MW01013285

NCLEX-PN® 101:

How To Pass!

Second Edition

NCLEX-PN® 101:

How To Pass!

Second Edition

Loretta Manning, MSN, RN, CS, GNP
President, I CAN Publishing®, Inc.
2650 Chattahoochee Drive, Suite 100
Duluth, Georgia 30097

Sylvia Rayfield, MN, RN, CNS
Board Chairwoman
Sylvia Rayfield & Associates, Inc.®
Pensacola, Florida

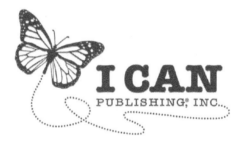

I CAN Publishing®, Inc. ◆ Duluth, GA
www.icanpublishing.com

Technical Assistance: Jennifer Robinson, Duluth, GA
and Mary Jo Zazueta, Traverse City, MI
Cartoon Illustrations: C.J. Miller, RN, Washington, IA
And Teresa Davidson, Greensboro, NC
Cover Design: Teresa Davidson, Greensboro, NC

© 2014 by I CAN Publishing®, Inc.

All rights reserved. No part of this book may be used or reproduced or transmitted in any form or by any means, electronic or mechanical, including photocopying, recording, or by an information storage and retrieval system without written permission from I CAN Publishing®, Inc. except for the inclusion of brief quotations in a review.

Printed in the United States of America
ISBN: 978-0-9903542-0-8
Library of Congress Control Number: 2014940253

Nursing procedures and practices described in this book should be applied by the nurse, or health-care practitioner, under appropriate supervision according to established professional standards of care. These standards should be used with regard to the unique circumstances that apply in each practice situation. Every effort has been taken to validate and confirm the accuracy of information presented and to describe generally accepted practices. However, the authors, editors, and publisher cannot accept any responsibility for errors or omissions or for consequences from application of the information in this book and make no warranty, express or implied, with respect to the contents of this book.

Every effort has been exerted by the authors and publisher to ensure that drug selection and dosage set forth in this text are in accord with current recommendations and practice at the time of publication. However, in view of ongoing research, the constant flow of information relating to government regulations, drug therapy, and drug reactions, the reader is urged to check the manufacturer's information on the package insert of each drug for any change in indications and dosage and for added warnings and precautions. This is particularly important when the recommended agent is a new or infrequently used drug.

This book is written to be used as a test question review book for the NCLEX-PN® examination. It is not intended for use as a primary resource for procedures, treatments, medications, or to serve as a complete textbook for nursing care.

Copies of this book may be obtained directly from:

I CAN Publishing®, Inc.
2650 Chattahoochee Drive, Suite 100
Duluth, GA 30097
770-495-2488
Web Site: www.icanpublishing.com

CONTENTS

Contributors   vii

Acknowledgments   ix

The Big Difference   xi

The NCLEX-PN® 101: HOW TO PASS! . . . .*xiii*

Prelude . . . .*xv*

What If You Knew . . . .*xvi*

Preparation for Success! . . . .*xvii*

Understanding What is Necessary to Know! . . . .*xviii*

NCLEX-PN® Exam . . . .*xix*

Blocks to Critical Thinking . . . .*xx*

How to be a Successful Thinker and Test Taker . . . .*xxi*

TEST-TAKING STRATEGIES

Steps to Success 1

Practice Answering Test Questions 2

Hot Tips to Decrease Stress and Improve Success 7

Let's Get Started 9

Alternate Exam Items "SAFETY" 11

"AIDES" in Answering Questions on Pharmacology 19

CHAPTER ONE   **THE PRE-TEST**

Questions 21

Category Analysis 29

Answers & Rationales 31

CHAPTER TWO   **SAFE AND EFFECTIVE CARE ENVIRONMENT: COORDINATED CARE**

Nursing Activities and Questions 42

Answers & Rationales 47

CHAPTER THREE   **SAFE AND EFFECTIVE CARE ENVIRONMENT: SAFETY AND INFECTION CONTROL**

Nursing Activities and Questions 54

Answers & Rationales 59

CHAPTER FOUR   **HEALTH PROMOTION AND MAINTENANCE**

Nursing Activities and Questions 66

Answers & Rationales 71

CHAPTER FIVE   PSYCHOSOCIAL INTEGRITY

Nursing Activities and Questions........................78

Answers & Rationales 84

CHAPTER SIX   PHYSIOLOGICAL INTEGRITY:
BASIC CARE AND COMFORT

Nursing Activities and Questions........................92

Answers & Rationales 97

CHAPTER SEVEN   PHYSIOLOGICAL INTEGRITY:
PHARMACOLOGICAL THERAPIES

Nursing Activities and Questions........................104

Answers & Rationales 109

CHAPTER EIGHT   PHYSIOLOGICAL INTEGRITY:
REDUCTION OF RISK POTENTIAL

Nursing Activities and Questions........................116

Answers & Rationales 121

CHAPTER NINE   PHYSIOLOGICAL INTEGRITY:
PHYSIOLOGICAL ADAPTATION

Nursing Activities and Questions........................128

Answers & Rationales 133

CHAPTER TEN   POST-TEST

Questions 139

Category Analysis Post-Test..........................153

Answers & Rationales 156

CHAPTER ELEVEN BONUS POST-TEST

Questions....................................169

Category Analysis Bonus Post-Test 175

Answers & Rationales 177

CONTRIBUTORS

Carol Anne Baker, BSN, MBA/HA, RN
Director of Nursing Services
Sentara Nursing Center
Virginia Beach, Virginia

Darlene Franklin, MSN, RN
Assistant Professor of Nursing Emeritus
Whitson-Hester School of Nursing
Tennessee Technological University
Cookeville, Tennessee

Melissa Geist, EdD, APRN-BC, CNE
Associate Professor of Nursing
Whitson-Hester School of Nursing
Tennessee Technological University
Interim Dean, College of Interdisciplinary Studies
Associate Professor of Nursing
Tennessee Technological University
Cookeville, Tennessee

Sylvia McDonald, RN, MEd, MSN
Consultant
I CAN Publishing®, Inc.
Sylvia Rayfield & Associates, Inc.®
Duluth, GA

Paula McNelis, RN, BSN
LPN Coordinator
Horry Georgetown Technical Community College
Myrtle Beach, South Carolina

Tina Rayfield, RN, BS, PA-C, MSN
President
Sylvia Rayfield & Associates, Inc.®
Pensacola, Florida

ACKNOWLEDGMENTS

We give our sincere appreciation to all of our contributors who helped make this book possible.

We want to thank Jennifer Robinson for her great organizational skills, patience, sense of humor, and always ready to jump through hoops to make this book a reality. I might add she did it with a smile and we love you for this, Jennifer!

We want to thank our families and friends who support all of our endeavors. A very special thank you to my mother, Juanita Shera, who has encouraged me all of my life and has always supported me in both my personal and professional life. I want to thank my husband, Randy Manning, who is always by my side with love and support. I want to thank Erica, our daughter, for all of her love and support and willingness to help with the final details of this book. Thank you to Burger for your support, love, and special ability to assist with details.

Thank you to all of you students, graduates, and faculty who continue to read and study our books! Without each of you, we would not be writing any of these acknowledgments!

THE BIG DIFFERENCE

We care enough to give you "**COURAGE**" to succeed!

C omparable to NCLEX®

O rganized around activities in NEW NCLEX-PN® Test Plan

U CAN do this and be successful!

R ationales for correct and incorrect answers

A ssociate and link questions with memory techniques to help you succeed!

G ive yourself a break every hour and review what you just studied!

E liminate studying "*nice to know*" and focus on "*need to know*" information!

NCLEX-PN® 101: HOW TO PASS!

This book has been written to transform your thinking from thinking like a student nurse to a graduate nurse. The items have been written succinctly to mimic the computer adaptive test. Plus, we have made a distinct effort to save as much paper (and consequently as many trees) as possible.

Our objective is to help you be successful and PASS by providing the latest information on the NCLEX-PN® exam. The exam as reflected by the test plan published by the National Council of State Boards of Nursing was updated in the 2012 Practice Analysis and will be implemented for the April 2014 exams. The chapter titles and items in this edition reflect these changes.

The butterfly on the cover of this book exemplifies your transformation and signifies your ability to spread your wings and fly through the NCLEX-PN® successfully after completing this book.

We will help you replace

F	False		**F**	Feel confident
E	Expectations of failing		**A**	Activities on NCLEX®
A	Appearing	WITH	**I**	I CAN DO IT!
R	Real		**T**	Thinking skills
			H	Help with study plan

*Remember, "It is ok to have butterflies in your stomach,
as long as they fly **In Formation**."*

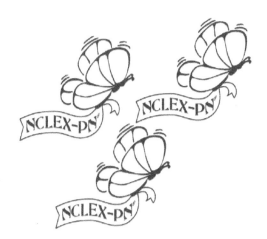

*The book has been written to get these butterflies to fly **"In Formation!"***

Prelude

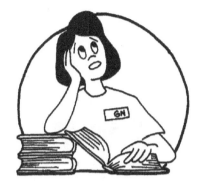

✦ What if you've just graduated from nursing school?

✦ What if you've just applied to take the NCLEX® exam?

✦ What if you have 50,000 pages of notes, tape recordings, and nursing books, and you don't have a clue as to where to start?

✦ What if you just need help?

Then ...

Read on ...

What if you knew—

✦ How to focus—not freak out

✦ Proven NCLEX® test-taking strategies

✦ How the NCLEX® is organized

✦ How to determine your own study needs

✦ What the questions look like on the computer exam

✦ That test questions in this book are organized around the most current NCLEX-PN® Test Plan

NCLEX-PN® PREPARATION FOR SUCCESS!

N	National	→	N	NCLEX® style questions
C	Council	→	C	Competencies (minimal)
L	Licensure	→	L	Level of Nursing Practice
E	Exam	→	E	Easy ways to review needs
X	Exam	→	X	Xactly what is necessary to know

P ractice Questions and Answers with rationales

N ew Test Plan reviewed with nursing activities

Reference: *National Council State Boards of Nursing*, 2012. Copyright © 2013 National Council of State Boards of Nursing, Inc. (NCSBN), *2012 LPN/VN Practice Analysis: Linking the NCLEX-PN® Examination to Practice*. 2014 NCLEX-PN® Test Plan.

All gray boxes at the beginning of Chapters 2-9 are interpreted from this *Practice Analysis*. We want to extend our appreciation to the NCSBN for their hard work in compiling this data.

PASS THE NCLEX-PN® *by*

UNDERSTANDING WHAT IS NECESSARY TO KNOW!

What is the NCLEX-PN®?
Answer: An exam administered by state boards of nursing who are mandated to protect the public from unsafe nursing practice. Each state board of nursing has a responsibility to regulate the practice of nursing in its respective state.

What is the purpose of the exam?
Answer: The NCLEX-PN® is to evaluate minimal **competency** to determine if you will be safe and effective. The exam will determine if you are competent at making clinical decisions.

How is the level of Nursing Practice determined? Level of thinking?
Answer: The National Council of State Boards of Nursing conducts a job analysis every 3 years to analyze the responsibilities of an entry level nurse. The exam is revised by the National Council based on study results. These results are outlined in the Test Plan and content and level of difficulty of exam items will reflect this study. The majority of items are written at the application or higher level of cognitive ability. For example, a medical surgical client undergoing a medical procedure may also have a mental illness and all factors must be considered in order to prepare the client for the procedure and to answer the item correctly.

What is a CAT Exam?
Answer: *CAT* is an acronym for *Computer Adaptive Test*. The candidate's response to the exam item directs the exam. The first few questions are important because they will move the candidate in the direction of difficulty based on these initial responses. If these initial questions are answered correctly, the computer progresses to a slightly more difficult question. If the questions are answered incorrectly, then the computer proceeds with a slightly easier question. The questions will be adapted to the ability of the candidate. The NCLEX-PN® Test Plan and the level of item difficulty are the framework for the exam.

X(Ex)actly, what is the bottom line information I need to know to be successful on the exam?
Answer: 1. There is a maximum of 5 hours to complete the exam. This includes the initial tutorial, an optional ten-minute break after the first two hours of testing, and an optional break after an additional 90 minutes of testing.

2. The exam includes a minimum of 85 questions with a maximum of 205 questions. There will be 15 questions used for validation purposes or experimental. These are being evaluated for future use on NCLEX-PN® exam and do not assist you or go against you.

3. Content – The gray boxes in front of each chapter in the book will outline the NCLEX® activities that will be evaluated on the NCLEX-PN®. The following page outlines the category of Client Needs and percentages represented on the exam.

NCLEX-PN® EXAM

The NCLEX-PN® exam is organized around the framework of "Client Needs." There are four categories of Client Needs and eight subcategories. This is published in the *National Council State Boards of Nursing, 2012 LPN/LVN Practice Analysis Linking the NCLEX-PN® Examination to Practice. Implemented for 2014 NCLEX-PN®.*

- ➢ **Safe and Effective Care Environment:**
  - Coordinated Care   16–22%
  - Safety and Infection Control   10–16%

- ➢ **Health Promotion and Maintenance**   7–13%

- ➢ **Psychosocial Integrity**   8–14%

- ➢ **Physiological Integrity:**
  - Basic Care and Comfort   7–13%
  - Pharmacological Therapies   11–17%
  - Reduction of Risk Potential   10–16%
  - Physiological Adaptation   7–13%

Several processes are also integrated throughout the NCLEX-PN® exam. These include the following: nursing process, caring, communication and documentation, and teaching/learning principles.

After the research is completed, the "nursing activities" become the "backbone" of the NCLEX-PN® exam. These are divided into the four categories of "Client Needs" as outlined above.

You will find a list of our interpretation of the "nursing activities" at the beginning of each chapter, except the Pre-Test, Post-Test, and Bonus Test.

Reference: National Council State Boards of Nursing, 2012. Copyright © 2013 National Council of State Boards of Nursing, Inc. (NCSBN), 2012 LPN/VN Practice Analysis: Linking the NCLEX-PN® Examination to Practice. 2014 NCLEX-PN® Test Plan.

BLOCKS TO CRITICAL THINKING

P *"Poor me" attitude (shut off your negative tape recorder and remember* The Little Engine That Could: **I CAN, I CAN, I CAN!!***)*

I *Inappropriate preparation (don't worry about old notes and tapes; use questions to determine your needs).*

T *"Too much work, too little time" (passing this exam is an investment in your future; PRIORITIZE).*

S *Spending too much time griping (use your time to practice questions).*

How to be a Successful
THINKER AND TEST TAKER

T *Take time to think through situations!*

H *Help focus on what is most important in the stem of the question!*

I *Identify exactly what the question is asking.*

N *No need to focus on information not needed to answer question.*

K *Knowledge must not just be memorized, but applied and / or analyzed.*

*S*urround yourself with
people who respect you and
treat you well.

—Claudia Black

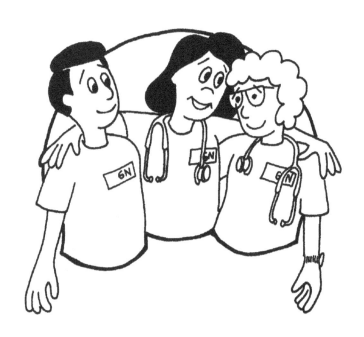

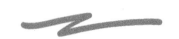

Supportive people give you strength. It's hard to think with people putting you down.

Remember ...

If you think you can do it—you can!

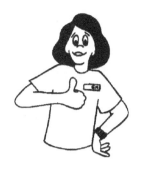

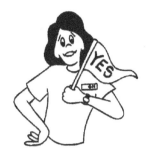

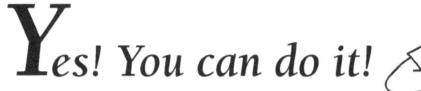

*Y*es! You can do it!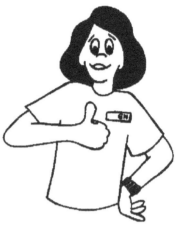

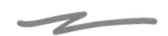

*N*ow let's get started on how you can be successful on the NCLEX-PN®!

STEPS TO SUCCESS

R Remove options prior to reading by covering distracters.

E Evaluate question by reading carefully, underlining key words, and develop pool of answers.

A Always review each option 1 at a time and decide if it is a possible answer.

D Decide on best answer.

S Study 1 hour a day reviewing questions and 1 hour reviewing content you missed.

A Application/Analysis are evaluated versus basic knowledge.

N Note tubes, graphs, images may be on exam.

S Standardized exams are predominantly multiple choice.

W Watch out for alternate exam items (Refer to "SAFETY").

E Eliminate any negative thoughts; replace with "I CAN do this!"

R Review content that you are missing in the questions in this book. (Reference *Nursing Made Insanely Easy!* by Manning and Rayfield.)

PRACTICE ANSWERING TEST QUESTIONS

Step 1

"Remove options prior to reading by covering DISTRACTERS."

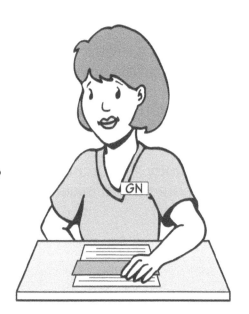

Sample Question:

What is the priority plan for the nursing student who is preparing for the NCLEX-PN® and is in a state of panic?

➤ You can't be DISTRACTED if options are covered.

➤ We do not want you to be DISTRACTED—so cover the DISTRACTERS with your hand, a 5x7 card, etc.

➤ Try to answer the question in your head. USE YOUR BRAIN. IT'S THE ONLY THING YOU CAN TRUST!

I CAN Publishing®, INC.

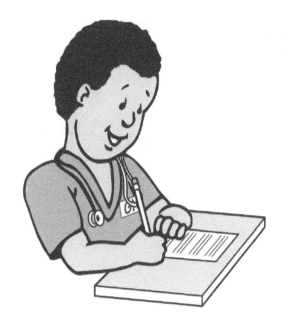

Step 2

"Evaluate questions by reading carefully, underlining key words, and developing a pool of answers."

What is the **priority plan** for the nursing student who is **preparing** for the **NCLEX-PN**® and is in a **state of panic**?

Pool of possible answers:

①　Reviewing volumes of notes from school.

②　Memorizing flash cards.

③　Buying 3 review books to study.

④　Panicking.

⑤　Praying.

⑥　Denying reality by going to a party!

If you practice by designing the structure for the answers in your head prior to reviewing the possible answers, your confidence will also increase! When you go into take the NCLEX®, do not look for just 1 correct answer. This is about making a decision regarding the best that you have to select from.

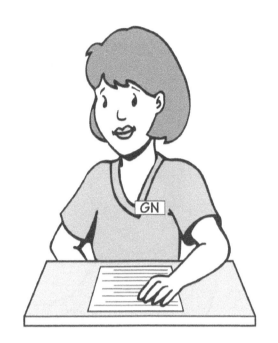

Step 3

"Always review each option one at a time and decide if it is a possible answer."

What is the **priority plan** for the nursing student who is **preparing** for the **NCLEX-PN**® and is in a **state of panic**?

①   Memorize and review volumes of facts from school.   *possible*

②   Practice from question books that you have already reviewed.   *possible*

③   Review notes from school.   *possible*

④   Begin by understanding the standards that are on the revised NCLEX-PN® Test Plan.   *yes*

Option #1 is a potential answer since this is how I survived in nursing school. OK, I need to be truthful . . . there were times I did not feel as if I was going to survive nursing school with all of these volumes of facts and facts and facts. Option #2 is a potential answer, but I am not certain it is a good idea to keep reviewing the same questions over and over again. I believe that would result in memorizing the questions versus processing them. Option #3 is just so overwhelming! I am not certain if I can even begin. I honestly do NOT like this option. Option #4 sounds like a great option, but I am not certain if I understand what these standards are or even where to go to find out this information.

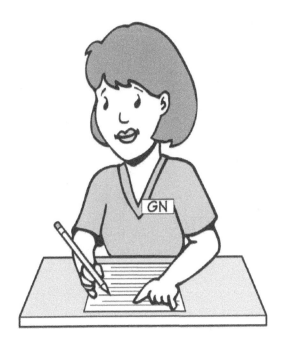

Step 4

"Decide on best answer."

Answer:

④ Option #4 is correct. Prior to initiating any study plan, the student must understand what standards are currently on the revised NCLEX-PN®, so you can work "smarter versus harder". These will be in gray boxes in the beginning of chapters 2 – 9. Options #1 and #3 are similar and both focus on past information. Option #2 is incorrect because this plan promotes memorization versus thinking and problem solving.

Congratulations on selecting the correct answer! Congratulations even if you did not select the correct answer because you are on the path to success! This entire book has been written within the framework of the NEW Test Plan which will be implemented April 1, 2014.

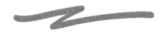

Step 5

"Study two hours a day: one hour reviewing questions and one hour reviewing content you missed."

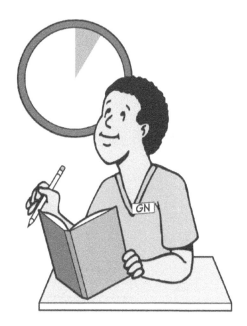

➤ Research has documented that the more questions practiced, the better the outcomes on the NCLEX®!

➤ Answer all the questions in this book and understand why you missed them.

➤ We recommend you answer approximately 1 question per minute.

➤ Answer all of the questions in each chapter prior to reviewing the answers. We want you to practice answering a specific number of questions during your study sessions without getting "immediate gratification."

➤ Looking at the answers after each question reinforces memorization. WE DO NOT WANT YOU TO MEMORIZE! This can result in additional anxiety since the test has been developed to evaluate your thinking and problem solving.

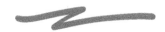

I CAN Publishing®, INC.

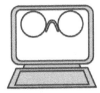

HOT TIPS to Decrease Stress and Improve Scores!

You can take the test in any state and practice in the state where you have applied for your license. You will have choices of dates, times, and test centers. You will be FINISHED WITHIN HOURS! The NCSBN currently contracts with Pearson Vue for administration of the NCLEX®. Pearson Vue has over 200 testing sites that administer the NCLEX®.

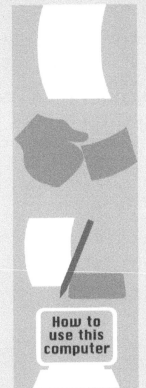

♥ You will get an authorization to test from your state board office. It's like American Express—"Don't leave home without it!"

♥ Don't leave home without your finger either because you will be fingerprinted and have your picture taken. You will need your signature and your picture identification for the testing center.

♥ You may be provided with lockers for your "stuff."

♥ You will be given a computer practice period with help on the equipment. There will be someone to help you get started on your computer—a warm-up time.

♥ The testing center will provide note boards and markers as you will not be allowed to take in any paper, books, food, drinks, purses, wallets, beepers, cell phones, guns, knives. *Security is very serious.*

♥ There will be a drop-down calculator for math calculations and a mouse for your use.

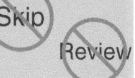

♥ There are a minimum of 85 questions and a maximum of 205. About 60% of test takers complete the exam in about 85 questions. DO NOT PANIC if you hit question #86! It means you have more time to demonstrate your intelligence.

85 to 205 questions

♥ You will have five (5) hours to complete the NCLEX-PN®. This is from start to finish, including warm-up time.

♥ You will not be able to skip a question or go back and review questions once you have left the screen. This is an advantage since many "changed" answers are wrong.

♥ There is no time limit per question, but **DO NOT SIT ON A QUESTION FOR MORE THAN TWO (2) MINUTES** or you may not have enough time in the five-hour limitation to answer enough questions to pass.

No more than 2 minutes per question

♥ If you don't have a clue as to the answer, pick any one.

Which response represents the best guess?
1. Alright!
2. Boy Howdy!
3. Cool!
4. Delightful!

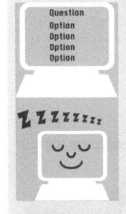

♥ The questions in this book look similar to the ones you will see on the computer screen.

♥ The computer offers you break times. Take time for breaks!

I CAN Publishing®, INC.

Let's Get STARTED!

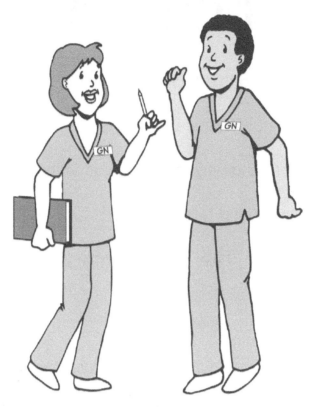

"The secret of getting ahead is getting started. The secret of getting started is breaking your complex, overwhelming tasks into small manageable tasks, and then starting on the first one." ~ MARK TWAIN

I CAN Memory Butterfly to help you fly **"In Formation!"** Memory techniques will be adapted in some of the rationales from *Nursing Made Insanely Easy!* by Manning and Rayfield. Visit www.icanpublishing.com or phone 770-495-2488 to purchase a complete book full of memory tools to help you be successful by remembering what is most IMPORTANT!

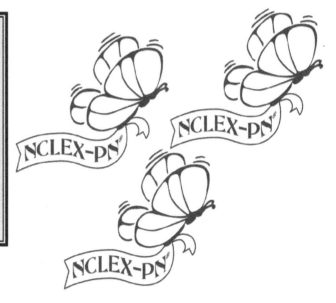

START NOW!

S Start by reviewing this book

T Thinking/Testing—Review Exam style

A Always understand why you miss a question

R Review answers and rationales

T Think "I CAN DO THIS!" and believe in yourself

N Note what questions you missed? Were they Safe and Effective Care Environment, Health Promotion, Psychosocial Integrity, Physiological Integrity? Use the Category Analysis, the Answers and Rationales, and Exam Grid.

O Once you have determined your study needs, use a good review book to refresh your memory on facts. We recommend *Nursing Made Insanely Easy* and *Pharmacology Made Insanely Easy* by Loretta Manning and Sylvia Rayfield, I CAN Publishing®, Inc. (770-495-2488 or www.icanpublishing.com). We also recommend *Illustrated Study Guide for the NCLEX-PN®* by JoAnn Zerwekh, Publisher Elsevier. www.elsevierhealth.com.

W Watch which questions you are answering correctly and positively reinforce your success! Review the alternate exam items beginning on next page. Remind yourself, "I CAN do this!"

ALTERNATE EXAM ITEMS

S Select all that apply (Multiple–response)

A Area select "Hot Spots" and click mouse
All types may include multimedia, such as charts,
tables, graphs, sounds, and video
Auditory–Use headphones to listen to an audio clip

F Fill-in-the-blanks/calculations

E Evaluate ordered response/Drag and Drop

T Test questions are multiple choice (majority)

Y Yes, thinking/decision making are keys to success

*Note: Any item format may include multi-media, chart
exhibits, tables, graphs, images, etc.*

ALTERNATE EXAM ITEMS

In this section, we will review the individual alternate exam items and review strategies to assist you in answering these exam items successfully.

S = Select All That Apply

Which nursing actions indicate the LPN / VN understands how to safely provide care for a client with Clostridium Difficile? **(Select all that apply.)**

- ☐ 1. The LPN / VN washes hands with alcohol antiseptic solution.
- ☐ 2. The LPN / VN instructs clients to share bedside tables.
- ☐ 3. The LPN /VN wears a mask when providing care to client.
- ☐ 4. The LPN / VN gowns when entering the client's room.
- ☐ 5. The LPN / VN wears gloves when providing care to client.

➤ **M** Mouse will be used to click on the box in front of the answers.

➤ **O** Organize these in your mind as mini "true and false questions."

➤ **U** Usually 5 or 6 options are provided. There is a box in front of each answer.

➤ **S** Stem – after it will read "Select all that apply."

➤ **E** Evaluate all correct responses when determining answers.

In order to answer this question correctly, it is imperative that you understand the appropriate precautions for a client with Clostridium Difficile which is contact precautions. Based on these precautions, the correct answers are options #4 and #5. Option #1 is not correct for Clostridium Difficile. Alcohol is not sporicidal. Clostridium Difficile requires contact isolation precautions. Option #2 is not correct for this isolation precaution. Equipment and tables should not be shared between clients. Option #3 is not a part of this standard. This would be necessary if the client was in droplet, airborne, or protective isolation (neutropenic precautions).

I CAN Publishing®, INC.

A = Area select "Hot Spots" and click mouse

While assessing cranial nerve 11, what part of the body would the nurse ask the client to move?

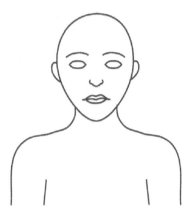

The question asks you to point to a location on an image (graphic) or table. This category of question has been developed to evaluate your understanding of physiology, physical assessment, and nursing content. This question is asking you to point to a part of the body that you would assess to evaluate cranial nerve number 11. In this question, you need to understand and know the 12 cranial nerves. *Nursing Made Insanely Easy*, by Loretta Manning and Sylvia Rayfield, has a great learning strategy that will help you remember these cranial nerves forever and with minimal effort!

In order to answer this question, use the mouse of the computer, move the cursor to the location you think is correct. Then, left-click the mouse. Review to make certain you have the location you want. At this time you can enter your answer by clicking the NEXT (N) button.

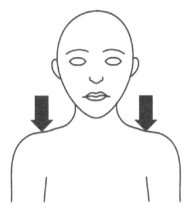

Answer: Cranial nerve 11 is the spinal accessory.

F = Fill-in-the-blanks – Enter the answer

The LPN/VN is providing care for a client who is on a clear liquid diet. He has an IV infusing at 120 mL per hour and it has infused for 5 hours. He consumed the following at this breakfast:

8 oz Tea
1 cup of jello
4 oz. Apple juice
½ cup of soup

Calculate and record the client's fluid intake in milliliters.

[   ] mL

Calculate the client's intake from the question. It is important for you to pay close attention to the unit of measure that is required in the answer. The question is asking to calculate the intake in milliliters.

The computer will have a drop-down calculator to assist you with the math. It can be found on the bottom of the right side of the computer screen. The mouse can be used to click on the numbers or functions necessary to complete the calculation. Remember "/" is division.

Begin answering the question by calculating the fluid intake from the IV.

120 mL x 5 = **600 mL** of fluid intake

Then progress to adding in the po intake. Begin by converting cups into ounces. One cup of fluid is equivalent to 8 ounces. The next step is to convert ounces into milliliters. One ounce = 30 milliliters.

8 oz Tea x 30 = **240**
1 cup jello = 8 oz x 30 = **240**
4 oz Apple juice x 30 = **120**
½ cup of soup = 4 oz x 30 = **120**

Then add the IV intake and po intake to get the **final answer.**

    600
+   720
  [1,320] mL

The computer mouse will move the cursor into the text box. Left-click on cursor. Type in the number representing the appropriate fluid intake. Only type in the no. Do not type in the units of measure. The only thing that goes in the box is the number.

Other examples of fill-in-the blank questions may be to establish priorities or determine a series of steps for specific nursing actions or interventions for a specific procedure, nursing care, etc.

E = Evaluate ordered response / Drag and Drop

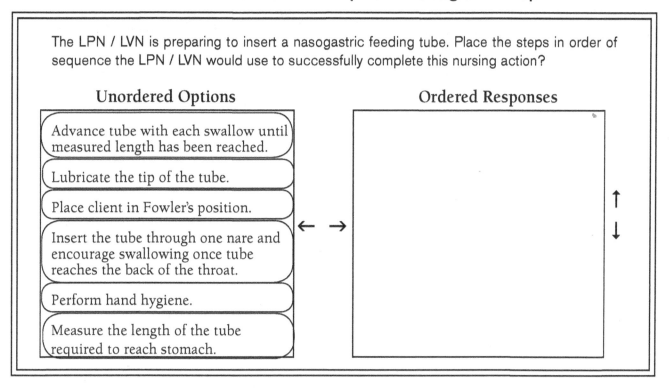

The LPN / LVN is preparing to insert a nasogastric feeding tube. Place the steps in order of sequence the LPN / LVN would use to successfully complete this nursing action?

Unordered Options

- Advance tube with each swallow until measured length has been reached.
- Lubricate the tip of the tube.
- Place client in Fowler's position.
- Insert the tube through one nare and encourage swallowing once tube reaches the back of the throat.
- Perform hand hygiene.
- Measure the length of the tube required to reach stomach.

← →

Ordered Responses

↑
↓

Strategy for answering this question is to remember "ICE". Remember the procedure should be as slick as ice!

I   INFECTION CONTROL

C   CLIENT Preparation

E   EQUIPMENT

Always begin with the end in mind before tackling any questions. A football team would NEVER begin to play without a plan! Nor should a nursing student who is either taking test questions or even initiating nursing care at the bedside begin without a plan. This will increase your confidence during this process!

I   Infection control is where we must start and stop! Always think hand washing and prevent infection.

C   Client preparation is the next step. Preparation may include appropriate positioning of the client, measuring the tube, lubricating, and then the procedure.

E   Equipment then should be the next part of the process. Appropriate procedure for this insertion must be considered.

Click on an option and drag it to the box on the right in order to begin placing the options in the correct order. Another approach for placing the options in the correct order is to move the left column to the right column by highlighting the option and clicking the arrow key that points to the column on the right. The order can also be rearranged in the right column by using the arrow keys pointing up and down.

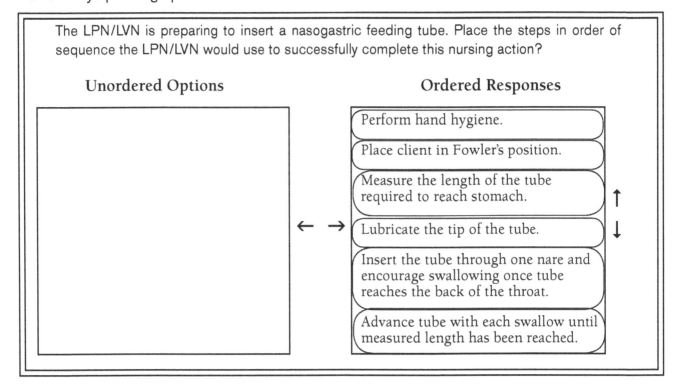

The LPN/LVN is preparing to insert a nasogastric feeding tube. Place the steps in order of sequence the LPN/LVN would use to successfully complete this nursing action?

Unordered Options

Ordered Responses

Perform hand hygiene.

Place client in Fowler's position.

Measure the length of the tube required to reach stomach.

Lubricate the tip of the tube.

Insert the tube through one nare and encourage swallowing once tube reaches the back of the throat.

Advance tube with each swallow until measured length has been reached.

I CAN Publishing®, INC.

T = Test questions are multiple choice (majority)

Y = Yes, critical thinking/decision making - keys to success

We have already reviewed the *"Steps to Success"* in answering multiple choice questions which represent the majority of the questions. The strategies necessary for these were outlined in *"READS ANSWER"*. What we still need to do is to review what is involved in critical thinking for the LPN / LVN. The word *"CRITICAL"* will assist you with this process and make it bottom line and easy to remember!

C   Criteria needs to be established to evaluate options / distracters

R   Relationships and patterns should be established

I   Identify what is most important in the question and options

T   Transfer knowledge from one situation to another

I   Identify the problem

C   Choices and / or course of nursing action must be discriminated between

A   Apply knowledge

L   Look and observe

R   Remove options prior to reading by covering distracters

E   Evaluate question by reading carefully, underlining key words, and developing a pool of answers

A   Always review each option 1 at a time and decide if it is a possible answer

D   Decide on best answer

What would be the highest priority for a client 72 hours after having 2nd degree burns to 20% of his body in the lower abdominal area and both legs?

1. We will not review options here, so we can begin thinking on our own.

2. Let's evaluate the question for key words and develop a pool of answers. The key words are as follows: **highest priority, 72 hours, 2nd degree burns, to lower abdominal area and legs.**

3. A pool of information for potential answers may include airway (Isn't this always a priority from a testing strategy?), nutrition, fluid, discomfort, psychological issues including image and / or anxiety. I am sure the list could go on and on, but for the exam we need to focus on the priorities.

4. Now it is time to evaluate each option one at a time, so let's get started!

1. Airway   *yes, this is included in our pool of possible answers.*

2. Body Image   *yes, this is a possibility.*

3. Fluid & Electrolytes   *yes, this is definitely a possibility.*

4. Pain   *yes, this is important, but probably not as important as fluid and electrolytes.*

Answer: Option #4 is correct. This client is 72 hours post burns and is high risk for major pain. Option #1 is incorrect since the burns are on lower extremities and airway is not currently involved or affected. Option #2 is not a priority within 72 hours. (*Always remember physiology is a priority over psychology.*) Option #3 would have been an answer prior to 72 hours. At 72 hours, however, the F & E should be stable.

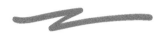

"AIDES"—

A STRUCTURE FOR ANSWERING QUESTIONS ON PHARMACOLOGY

A Action, assessment, administration, accuracy of order or "prescription"

I Identify priority plan, Interactions

D Desired outcome

E Evaluate client's response to medication. Education reinforcement regarding meds.

S Safety (identification, order abbreviations, expiration, compatibility, start and monitor peripheral IV)

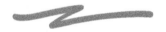

CHAPTER 1
The Pre-Test

*Tenderness and kindness are not signs
of weakness and despair, but manifes-
tations of strength and resolution.*
—Kahlil Gibran

✔ About this test ...

This 60-item test will help you begin to pinpoint your study needs.

FOR BEST RESULTS:

☞ Complete the entire Pre-Test. Do NOT look in the back of the book for the answers until you have completed the exam.

☞ Spend a few minutes analyzing the questions you have missed. Use the test worksheet and Category Analysis to help determine your study needs. Once you determine your weak area(s), spend the next hour studying this content using a good review book as a guide.

REMEMBER THAT MISTAKES ARE A WAY OF GROWING—
BE GENTLE WITH YOURSELF!
"The reason that angels can fly is that they take themselves so lightly."
—G. K. Chesterson

These activities are taken from the *Reference: National Council State Boards of Nursing*, 2012. Copyright © 2013 National Council of State Boards of Nursing, Inc. (NCSBN), *2012 LPN/VN Practice Analysis: Linking the NCLEX-PN® Test Plan.*

TOMORROW—

☞ Skip to the chapter in this book that asks questions on the area of your biggest identified weakness.

☞ Take the test from this chapter and note the questions that you missed. Spend the next hour studying this content. ETC! ETC! ETC!

1.1 Which one of these clients should be assessed first following shift report?

① A primipara client, with an oxytocin infusion, who delivered an 8 lb. 4 oz. daughter 45 minutes ago.
② A primigravida client who is presenting in the last trimester with a small amount of painless, bright red blood and fetal heart rate (FHR)–130 beats/min with good variability.
③ Multipara client, one hour after a precipitate delivery, presents with a BP–98/62, HR–102, with pale and clammy skin. Fundus is firm and midline.
④ A postpartum client who delivered 24 hours ago, is presenting with a temperature of 100°F and in last 24 hours diuresed 2000 ml.

1.2 The LPN is administering medications to a group of clients. Which one of these medication administrations should the charge nurse intervene with immediately?

① Lispro (Humalog) insulin to a client when the breakfast tray arrives.
② Metoprolol (Lopressor) prior to surgery for a client with pheochromocytoma.
③ Propranolol (Inderal) for a client with hyperthyroidism.
④ Metformin HCL (Glucophage) to a client with a creatinine of 3.8mg/dL.

1.3 Which of these actions by an unlicensed assistive personnel (UAP) for a client with mitral insufficiency need intervention from the nurse due to not following the standard of care for this medical condition?

① Encourages client to drink fluids hourly.
② Performs frequent oral hygiene.
③ Reports T–101.9°F.
④ Recommends client to conserve energy and not get up frequently.

1.4 Which one of these clients should be assessed immediately after shift report?

① A client who has decreased bowel sounds on the first post-op day following a GI surgery.
② A client who is complaining of pain at the site of a liver biopsy one hour after procedure.
③ A client with pain in the right lower abdominal quadrant and is lying on the side with knees flexed.
④ A client who is experiencing a sudden relief from pain that was in the right lower abdominal quadrant.

1.5 Which statement made by the client with a spinal cord injury, who has just been transferred to a rehabilitation facility, indicates client needs additional information?

① "After rehabilitation I hope to return to my career."
② "After rehabilitation I may be able to achieve more control of my bladder."
③ "Rehabilitation will assist me in learning how to optimize my independence."
④ "During rehabilitation I will learn how to regain all of my motor functions."

1.6 A client with type 1 Diabetes Mellitus is seeing the nurse to review foot care. What would be a priority to include when reinforcing the discharge teaching plan the RN initiated?

① Examine feet once per week for redness, blisters, and abrasions.
② Apply lotion to dry feet, especially between the toes.
③ Avoid hot-water bottles and heating pads.
④ Dry feet vigorously after each bath.

1.7 The nurse notes many bruises in various stages of healing on the abdomen and bilateral legs on a pregnant client and some complaints of headaches. Vital signs are: BP–124/88, HR–80 BPM, RR–20/min, and FHR–128. Which of these responses would be the most appropriate?

① "You may have more accidents now that you are pregnant."
② "Tell me about your headaches and the frequency."
③ "Does your partner abuse you?"
④ "Do you have any concerns regarding your pregnancy?"

1.8 What is the priority of care for a client who is experiencing a manic episode and starting to become combative?

① Assist the client to the recreation room for a game of pool.
② Escort client to a quiet room with no other people or activities occurring.
③ Encourage client to verbalize thoughts and feelings.
④ Set firm limits on client's behavior and expectations.

1.9 What are the appropriate nursing actions for a client with undiagnosed abdominal pain? *Select all that apply.*

① Give client sips of water.
② Apply heat on the abdomen.
③ Maintain client on bed rest.
④ Administer morphine for acute pain.
⑤ Assess intake and output

1.10 In caring for a client with GERD, which task would be most appropriate to assign to the unlicensed assistive personnel (UAP)?

① Position client with the head of the bed elevated after eating.
② Encourage client to express concerns about lifestyle modification.
③ Review the importance for eating small, frequent meals.
④ Encourage client to use pillows to elevate head of the bed.

1.11 An 85-year-old client cannot swallow the antibiotic tablet. Which is the priority action?

① Crush the tablets, dissolve in milk, and allow the client to swallow them.
② Notify the healthcare provider for a different order.
③ Ask the pharmacist if liquid is available in this medication.
④ Ask family members to coax the client to swallow the tablets.

1.12 The client diagnosed with congestive heart failure wakes in the middle of the night gasping and saying "I can't breathe!" Which would be the priority nursing action?

① Place the client in the supine position and suction airway.
② Elevate the head of the bed.
③ Administer oxygen per protocol at 4 L/minute.
④ Assess the client's lung sounds.

1.13 The client diagnosed with diabetes mellitus has been prescribed a Methyl Prednisolone Dose Pack. What would be most important for the nurse to monitor for the client taking this drug?

① Serum glucose.
② Hemoglobin.
③ Stools for occult blood.
④ Vital Signs.

1.14 The client's admitting vital signs as recorded by the registered nurse were documented as P–80, R–20, BP–170/90. Half hour later the vital signs are P–82, R–22, BP–190/100. What would be the priority nursing action?

① Notify the Charge RN of the change in vital signs.
② Wait 15 minutes and retake the BP.
③ Document the findings.
④ Ask the client if he salted his lunch.

1.15 During the orientation session for new LPNs / LVNs, the instructor reviewed calcium channel blockers. During the clinical evaluation on the medical unit, the LPN has a client that just received the first dose of Norvasc (amlodipine) an hour ago. Which of these assessments indicate the LPN understands how to evaluate the client response to this medication?

① Respiratory rate.
② Reflexes.
③ Temperature.
④ Blood pressure.

1.16 Which of these clients should the nurse assess immediately after shift report?

① A client complaining of dizziness after getting out of bed quickly.
② A client who just stopped talking and is slumped over in bed.
③ A client with a blood pressure of 110/76 and it was 120/84 two hours earlier.
④ A client with a heart rate of 90 BPM.

1.17 What would be the priority nursing action for a client diagnosed with diabetes mellitus who presents with confusion, shaking, and diaphoresis?

① Assess vital signs.
② Administer insulin as ordered.
③ Provide client with a glass of milk.
④ Notify the HCP.

1.18 A client on renal dialysis taking warfarin (Coumadin) has decided to take Gingko Biloba for memory loss. What is the priority action?

① Take the Gingko from the client and flush it down the toilet.
② Confirm that the Gingko has been successfully used by client with decreased memory loss.
③ Inform the RN of this client decision.
④ Explain that both drugs administered together may cause bleeding tendencies.

1.19 The client's medical record indicates that a client is allergic to penicillin. There is a new order to administer acyclovir (Zovirax). Which nursing action would be the priority?

① Hold the acyclovir (Zovirax) as there is an incompatibility with penicillin.
② Assess the client's BUN and creatinine prior to administering the drug.
③ Assess the client's temperature prior to administering the medication.
④ Notify the HCP of the allergy to penicillin.

1.20 The mother of a 21-year-old asks the Emergency Department nurse to identify the admitting diagnosis for her son. Which action is most important?

① Advise the mother of the admitting diagnosis and ask for the name of the family provider.
② Ask the RN to speak to the mother.
③ Tell the mother that her son is of age and the diagnosis cannot be revealed to her.
④ Inform the mother that confidentiality laws prevent the release of information.

1.21 Which of the following should be included in the process for changing a dressing on a newborn? *Select all that apply.*

① Wash hands thoroughly and apply sterile gloves.
② Utilize sterile bandaging and secure with paper tape.
③ Teach the care giver the process for changing the bandage.
④ Dispose of the old bandage in an appropriate receptacle.
⑤ Document the procedure as being a "clean dressing change".

1.22 An elderly client, who resides in an assisted living facility, has been experiencing some delusions in the lunch room and is asking for the "before meal pill." The armband is lost. What would be the most appropriate action prior to administering the medication?

① Ask the client to state name and administer the medication.

② Ask the client's roommate for the name prior to administering medication and replace the armband.

③ Ask the UAP for the name of the client.

④ Determine the client's identification by checking the chart for a photograph.

1.23 What is the priority nursing action for a post operative client who has been admitted with Clostridium Difficile?

① Clean hands with alcohol antiseptic hand wash.

② Place client in private room and wear gloves and gown during nursing care.

③ Place client in a room with a client who has MRSA.

④ Wear gloves and mask when in the client's room.

1.24 The 5' tall client that weighs 179 pounds is to receive an I.M. injection of Bicillin. Which size needle should be selected for use?

① 20 gauge, 3 inch needle.

② 21 gauge, 1 to 1½ inch needle.

③ 25 gauge, 1 to 1½ inch needle.

④ 25 gauge 5/8 inch needle.

1.25 A 32-year-old pregnant client reporting episodes of rapid breathing, air hunger and tingling has an oxygen saturation reading of 97%. Which would be the appropriate nursing actions? *Select all that apply.*

① Assist the client to a high-Fowler's position.

② Reassess the client's O_2 saturation reading.

③ Administer oxygen @ 4 L/minute per protocol.

④ Turn the client to the left side and apply oxygen @ 1 L/minute per protocol.

⑤ Notify the healthcare provider of the assessment and nursing actions.

1.26 A 62-year-old client, who is 2nd day post-operative hip replacement, has an order to ambulate in the hall. The client expresses fear of getting out of the bed. What would be the appropriate nursing actions? *Select all that apply.*

① Ask an additional staff member to assist with the ambulation.

② Ask a family member to walk beside the client with a wheelchair in case this is needed.

③ Place a safety belt on the client that can be used to steady the walk.

④ Place a safety belt on both staff members for client to reach if needed.

⑤ Explain to the client the time and distance of the walk.

1.27 What is the priority of care for any client who experiences a seizure?

① Maintain a patent airway for the client.

② Assess vital signs prior to further action.

③ Ask the client if they can hear you.

④ Lower the client to the floor and wait for the seizure to be complete.

1.28 The daughter of a client who is in a nursing home reports that her mother has been beaten and has the bruises to prove it. Which actions should be taken? *Select all that apply.*

① Assess the client's bruises and ask her how she got them.

② Read the chart to determine if there are any recorded accident reports.

③ Speak to staff caring for the client and assess their reports.

④ File an incident report as reported by the daughter.

⑤ Call the police to report a possible assault and battery.

1.29 The client is to receive haloperidol (Haldol) 2mg injectable which is provided in 5mg/mL. How many mLs will be administered to this client? **Fill in the blank**.

_____ mLs

1.30 In planning the care of a client with an acute episode of Meniere's syndrome, the client should be taught which of the following?

   ① Adding salt to food.
   ② Avoiding sudden motion of the head.
   ③ Placing client in room closest to nurses' station.
   ④ Encouraging client to be up and walking in hall.

1.31 Which technique is best for obtaining a urine specimen for a culture and sensitivity from a client with an existing indwelling catheter?

   ① Clean the drain of the collecting bag with an antiseptic before filling the specimen container.
   ② Obtain the specimen from the drainage bag in the morning.
   ③ Using a sterile syringe with a small gauge needle, aspirate urine from the catheter port.
   ④ If the catheter has been in place for 48 hours, replace it before obtaining the specimen.

1.32 Which procedure indicates the nurse understands how to safely administer the DPT immunization to a 6-month-old child? The nurse administers the DPT:

   ① By mouth in three divided doses.
   ② As an IM injection into the gluteus maximus.
   ③ As an injection into the vastus lateralis.
   ④ As a deep Z track injection into the deltoid.

1.33 1000 ml 5% Dextrose in 0.45 Saline is to be administered IV over 8 hours using an infusion pump for an adult client. What is the correct rate setting on the IV pump? **Fill in the blank.** _____ mL / hour.

1.34 To promote safety, the nurse would implement which action in obtaining a blood specimen from a client who has been diagnosed with hepatitis B?

   ① Clean area with antiseptic solution.
   ② Wear a pair of clean gloves.

   ③ Apply pressure to site for 5 seconds.
   ④ Recap needle to avoid carrying exposed needle.

1.35 Organize these steps in chronological order with #1 being the first step for a client who is having a nasogastric tube removal.

   ① Assist the client into a semi-Fowler's position.
   ② Ask client to hold breath.
   ③ Assess bowel function by auscultation for peristalsis.
   ④ Flush tube with 10 mL of normal saline.
   ⑤ Withdraw the tube gently and steadily.
   ⑥ Monitor client for nausea, vomiting.

1.36 Which side effect of Trimethoprim-sulfamethoxazole (Bactrim) should the nurse instruct the client to report while taking this medication?

   ① Hypotonia.
   ① Loss of hearing.
   ③ Hypotension.
   ④ Urticaria.

1.37 Following an abdominal hysterectomy, which action would be a priority in preventing thrombophlebitis?

   ① Encourage support by using knee gatch.
   ② Decrease the fluid intake.
   ③ Encourage turning, coughing, and deep breathing every 2 hours.
   ④ Encourage active leg exercises and ambulation.

1.38 Following the death of a female client who is Muslim, the nurse should plan on providing the family with:

   ① A private room to gather the family for grieving.
   ② A Muslim wrap, preferably white, for the body.
   ③ Post-mortem care of the body by a female nurse.
   ④ Immediate referral to a crematory.

1.39 A 72-year-old client has an order for digoxin (Lanoxin) 0.25 mg po in the morning. The nurse reviews the following information: apical pulse = 68 BPM, respirations = 16/min., plasma digoxin level = 2.2 ng/mL. Based on this assessment, which nursing action is appropriate?

① Give the medication on time.

② Withhold the medication and notify the healthcare provider.

③ Administer epinephrine 1:1000 stat.

④ Check the client's blood pressure.

1.40 Which of these psychiatric clients should be evaluated first?

① Depressed client sitting on the floor rocking back and forth.

② Bipolar client pacing and clenching fist.

③ Psychotic client who is having a delusion that she is the Queen of England.

④ Schizophrenic client laughing and waving hands up in the air.

1.41 Which communication technique would be appropriate for a nurse to implement when caring for a client who has a hearing loss?

① Irrigate the ear with warm water to remove any wax obstruction.

② Always touch the client prior to speaking to him.

③ Encourage the client to purchase a hearing aid.

④ Stand in front of him and speak clearly and slowly.

1.42 What would be a priority in establishing a bladder retraining program?

① Provide a flexible schedule for the client to decrease anxiety.

② Schedule toileting on a planned time schedule.

③ Teach client intermittent self-catheterization.

④ Perform the Crede maneuver tid.

1.43 What is the correct procedure for obtaining a throat culture from a client with pharyngitis?

① Quickly rub a cotton swab over both tonsil and posterior pharynx areas.

② Obtain a sputum container for the client to use.

③ Swab the pharynx following irrigation with warm saline.

④ Hyperextend the client's head and neck for the procedure.

1.44 Which assessment would be most important for monitoring a client's state of hydration?

① Daily weights.

② I & O.

③ Skin tugor.

④ Characteristic of lips and mucous membranes.

1.45 A client discharged with sublingual nitroglycerin (Nitrostat) should be taught to:

① Take the medications 5 minutes after the pain has started.

② Stop taking the medication if a burning sensation is present.

③ Take the medication on an empty stomach.

④ Avoid abrupt changes in posture.

1.46 What is the priority nursing action prior to administering medications through a nasogastric tube?

① Consult a drug book regarding the recommendations for crushing each medication.

② Verify placement of the nasogastric tube in the abdomen through aspiration of gastric content.

③ Calculate the amount of water needed to dissolve each medication.

④ Clean out the pill crushers to get rid of any residue.

1.47 The psychiatric nurse is administering a depressed client doxepin hydrochloride (Sinequan) 75 mg po TID. This nurse should recommend a change in the client's therapy if which response occurs? The client:

① Refuses to speak and sits quietly in the room.

② Becomes excitable and develops tremors.

③ Refuses to eat breakfast.

④ Sleeps 18 hours a day.

1.48 Which nursing approach would be most appropriate to use while administering an oral medication to a 4-month-old child?

① Place medication in 45 mL of formula.
② Place medication in an empty nipple.
③ Place medication in a full bottle of formula.
④ Place in supine position and administer medication using a syringe.

1.49 Which clinical finding would be most appropriate for the LPN to report to the RN regarding the client taking furosemide (Lasix)?

① A weight loss of two pounds.
② Blood pressure change from 160/98 to 141/90.
③ An increase in urinary frequency.
④ A ringing in the ears.

1.50 Which sequence is correct when providing care for a client immediately prior to surgery?

① Administer preoperative medication, client signs operative permit, determine vital signs.
② Check operative permit for signature, advise the client to remain in bed, administer preoperative medication.
③ Remove client's dentures, administer preoperative medication, client empties bladder.
④ Verify client has been NPO. Client empties bladder, family leaves room.

1.51 A permanent demand pacemaker set at a rate of 72 beats per minute is implanted in a client for persistent third degree block. Which nursing assessment would indicate a pacemaker dysfunction?

① Pulse rate of 88 and irregular.
② Apical pulse rate regular at 68.
③ Blood pressure of 110/88 and pulse 78.
④ Tenderness at site of pacemaker implant.

1.52 A 24-year-old client who is 2 hours post delivery complains of nausea, being cold, and "feeling funny". Vital signs indicate a BP- 80/40, Pulse-120 beats per minute, Respirations-26 per minute. Which nursing action would be a priority?

① Assess for bleeding.
② Place in Trendelenberg position.
③ Contact the healthcare provider.
④ Administer PRN pain medication.

1.53 To complete an assessment of cranial nerve eleven, the client will be asked to:

① Move tongue.
② Identify a smell.
③ Read a Snellen chart.
④ Shrug both shoulders.

1.54 A round reddened quarter sized area is assessed on a bedridden client's coccyx area during the morning assessment. Which actions should be taken to improve skin integrity? *Select all that apply.*

① Clean and dry the area carefully.
② Place the client on a turn-every-2-hours plan.
③ Document the size, induration and skin condition.
④ Notify the provider for treatment options.
⑤ Place the client on appropriate isolation program.

1.55 In receiving morning report, the night nurse relates that the nurse on the previous shift forgot to sign off one of the charts; therefore, a space of a few lines was left for the nurse when returns to work. Which is the most appropriate action?

① Notify the supervisor prior to the night nurse leaving the unit.
② Call the nurse who forgot to chart to come in today to complete the chart.
③ Chart as usual leaving the blank space for the off duty nurse.
④ Notify the healthcare provider for direction.

1.56 The client has an order for 150 mL /hour of IV Ringer's lactate. The IV administration set delivers 10 gtts / mL. At what rate should the nurse set the infusion? **Fill in the blank.**
_____ gtts / minute

1.57 A fire develops in the unit at a long term care facility. The fire department is on the way, but due to thick smoke, the unit must be evacuated. Which client should the nurse evacuate first?

① A client who had a Cesarean section 45 minutes ago.
② A 30-year-old client who had an appendectomy 6 hours ago.
③ An 84-year-old client recovering from pneumonia.
④ An elderly client with COPD and is being maintained on IV fluids.

1.58 An adult client is to receive heparin sodium (Heparin) 5,000 units subcutaneously. Which technique indicates the nurse understood the information learned in orientation regarding the appropriate technique for the administration of this drug? The LPN:

① Gently massages the injection site.
② Administers the drug without aspirating.
③ Uses a one inch 18-20 gauge needle.
④ Administers the drug in the deltoid muscle.

1.59 List in chronological order how the nurse should put on the personal protection equipment?

① Gloves
② Gown
③ Goggles or face shield
④ Mask or respirator

1.60 The LPN is working for a home healthcare agency. Which finding, if observed, should be reported by the nurse? A client

① with an infected wound who allows cats to eat off the table.
② receiving intermittent oxygen therapy who has a spouse that smokes in the home.
③ with diabetes who has a bowl of candy sitting on the coffee table.
④ with COPD who sleeps in a recliner instead of a bed.

CATEGORY ANALYSIS – PRE-TEST

1. Coordinated Care
2. Pharmacological Therapies
3. Coordinated Care
4. Coordinated Care
5. Health Promotion
6. Health Promotion
7. Psychosocial Integrity
8. Psychosocial Integrity
9. Basic Care and Comfort
10. Coordinated Care
11. Pharmacological Therapies
12. Physiological Adaptation
13. Pharmacological Therapies
14. Reduction of Risk Potential
15. Pharmacological Therapies
16. Physiological Adaptation
17. Physiological Adaptation
18. Pharmacological Therapies
19. Pharmacological Therapies
20. Coordinated Care
21. Safety & Infection Control
22. Safety & Infection Control
23. Safety & Infection Control
24. Pharmacological Therapies
25. Physiological Adaptation
26. Safety & Infection Control
27. Reduction of Risk Potential
28. Coordinated Care
29. Pharmacological Therapies
30. Safety & Infection Control

31. Reduction of Risk Potential
32. Pharmacological Therapies
33. Pharmacological Therapies
34. Safety & Infection Control
35. Reduction of Risk Potential
36. Health Promotion
37. Basic Care and Comfort
38. Psychosocial Integrity
39. Physiological Adaptation
40. Psychosocial Integrity
41. Basic Care and Comfort
42. Basic Care and Comfort
43. Reduction of Risk Potential
44. Basic Care and Comfort
45. Health Promotion
46. Reduction of Risk Potential
47. Pharmacological Therapies
48. Health Promotion
49. Coordinated Care
50. Coordinated Care
51. Physiological Adaptation
52. Reduction of Risk Potential
53. Reduction of Risk Potential
54. Basic Care and Comfort
55. Coordinated Care
56. Pharmacological Therapies
57. Safety & Infection Control
58. Coordinated Care
59. Safety & Infection Control
60. Safety & Infection Control

DIRECTIONS

1. Determine questions missed by checking answers.
2. Write the number of the questions missed across the top line marked "item missed."
3. Check category analysis page to determine category of question.
4. Put a check mark under item missed and beside content.
5. Count check marks in each row and write the number in totals column.
6. Use this information to:
   • identify areas for further study.
   • determine which content test to take next.

We recommend studying content where most items are missed—then taking that content test.

Number of the Questions Incorrectly Answered

Pre-Test	Items Missed		Totals
Coordinated Care			3
Safety and Infection Control			3
Health Promotion and Maintenance			2
Psychosocial Integrity			2
Physiological Integrity: Physiological Adaptation			1
Physiological Integrity: Reduction of Risk			3
Physiological Integrity: Basic Care and Comfort			3
Physiological Integrity: Pharmacological Therapies			27

C O N T E N T

Items Missed (top line): 2 3 4 7 18 19 21 27 30 35 36 37 40 42 47 46 47 51 52 54 59

I CAN Publishing®, INC.

ANSWERS & RATIONALES

1.1 ③ Option #3 is correct since this client has vital signs that indicate bleeding and volume loss. The BP is low, the HR is fast and the color of the client is pale and skin temperature is clammy, a classic sign of a complication with bleeding. While the fundus is firm and midline, this just indicates that the client is not bleeding from a boggy fundus (uterine atony). There are two other causes of bleeding following delivery, which include retained placenta fragments and cervical lacerations. The bottom line is that even if you did not know the cause of the bleeding the clinical presentation of the multipara client provides an excellent description of a client experiencing complications from bleeding. Option #1 is incorrect. There is no reason for this to be the priority when this is given to assist with uterine contractions to help minimize complications from bleeding. Option #2 is incorrect. The client may be presenting with placenta previa. Yes, the nurse would need to assess this client, but this would not be a priority over a client who is actively bleeding with vital sign changes as in option #3. This client in option #2 only has a small amount of bleeding and the FHR is within normal range (120–160 beats per minute) with a sign of good oxygenation (variability). Option #4 is incorrect since these would be considered expected clinical findings for a postpartum client 24 hours following delivery.

I CAN HINT: "LABOR" will also assist you in organizing some of the key complications that would need to be prioritized for the maternity clients.

Late decelerations = uteroplacental insufficiency (Fetal tachycardia or bradycardia or loss of variability) (Normal FHR: 120–160)

Abdominal pain that is described as sharp/board like = abruption placenta!! OR epigastric pain!

Blurred vision, headache = late signs of preeclampsia (PIH); bright-red bleeding that is painless (placenta previa); signs and symptoms of bleeding

perio **O**rbital edema, edema in fingers, proteinuria, hypertension = early signs of preeclampsia (PIH); oxytocin test positive (compared to the other findings, in this mnemonic this would be a low priority)

Reduction in the insulin requirements in the LAST trimester; reduction in fetal movement as pregnancy progresses; rupture of the membranes (premature or spontaneous)

1.2 ④ Option #4 is correct. Metformin HCL (Glucophage) may cause lactic acidosis. Since the creatinine is 3.8 mg/dL (*normal: 0.5–1.5 mg/dL*), metformin (Glucophage) should not be administered due to the risk of renal complications developing from lactic acidosis. The nurse needs to intervene, since the LPN should hold this medication and notify the healthcare provider (HCP) because the medication should not be administered if the serum creatinine is > 1.5 mg/dL. Options #1, #2, and #3 are correct for the identified clients, so there is no need for the charge nurse to intervene with the LPN regarding care. Option #1 is a rapid-acting insulin and should only be administered in the A.M. when food is available. Option #2 is necessary due to the hypertension these clients can develop; a result of this rare disorder of the adrenal medulla characterized by a tumor that secretes an excess of epinephrine and norepinephrine. An increase in these catecholamines produces vasoconstriction, with a precipitant increase in blood pressure, glycogenolysis, and cardiac workload. Option #3 would be necessary from the risk of tachycardia as a result of the increase in the thyroid hormones that may occur in hyperthyroidism.

 I CAN HINT: The NCLEX® activity that is being evaluated is *"Recognize limitations of self/others and seek assistance."* A way to organize this information is to reflect on the word "**STANDARDS**." As you are studying, this will assist you in remembering when the nurse will need to intervene due to inappropriate care. If these are being violated or not implemented, then the nurse does need to intervene, such as in the question above when a major complication of metformin HCL (Glucophage) is lactic acidosis and the creatinine is elevated. This presents a major risk to the client with the renal system. This is only one aspect of care, however, that would require intervention by the nurse. Refer to the mnemonic below to assist you with other clinical situations that may present a risk to the client if the nurse does not intervene.

Standard of care is not being followed.

The position is not correct for the procedure or post-op care.

Assessments indicate a complication and the UAP, LPN, or RN have not addressed the finding.

Not linking the lab finding(s) with the medication, nursing care, diagnostic procedure, etc. (like in this question).

Dietary/fluid and electrolyte needs for specific medical condition are being ignored.

Acute versus chronic: nurse is focusing and prioritizing inappropriately with a focus on chronic versus acute.

Reviewing client identity prior to providing care is not being followed.

Does not focus on the SAFETY for the client, such as infection control, room placement, med safety, etc.

Scope of practice is not being followed.

1.3 ① Option #1 is correct. The nurse would need to intervene with the UAP due to the extra fluids the UAP is providing the client. A client with mitral insufficiency may present with crackles in the lungs,

dyspnea, orthopnea, palpitations, possible diminished lung sounds, S_3 and/or S_4 sounds, systolic murmur, atrial fibrillation. With this disorder there is improper closure of the mitral valve allowing blood to flow backward (regurgitation). The nursing care includes fluid and sodium restriction. Refer to I CAN HINT for additional nursing care. Option #2 is incorrect. The client would need oral hygiene since the care would include limiting fluids. Option #3 is incorrect. This temperature would need to be reported, so there is no need for the nurse to intervene. Option #4 is incorrect, since this is part of the care for this client.

 I CAN HINT: "MITRAL" will assist you in remembering the priority nursing care for clients with mitral insufficiency.

Monitor current weight and note any changes.

Intake of fluid and sodium restricted.

To decrease preload—Thiazide (Hydrodiuril), loop (Lasix) diuretics, potassium-sparing diuretics (Aldactone).

Review hemodynamic monitoring. (Left-sided valve insufficiency. Increased pulmonary artery pressure and decreased cardiac output.)

Assess heart rate and rhythm for regularity and for a murmur.

Learn about foods high in potassium, such as potatoes, oranges, bananas, etc.

1.4 ④ Option #4 needs to be assessed immediately after report because this sudden relief of pain may indicate a rupture of the appendix. This now is a medical emergency and demands immediate intervention. Option #1 is an expected finding during this post-op period. Option #2 is also an expected finding following this procedure. Client needs to be comforted and assessed, but it is not a priority over option #4 who is an emergency. Option #3 is a concern and must be assessed, but option #4 is the emergency due to the potential rupture.

 I CAN HINT: When you assess any sudden relief of pain for a client who is presenting with appendicitis, this becomes a priority due to the risk for rupturing and all of the complications that go along with a rupture. Clinical decision-making is all about making the best decision with the options available. Remember, while they might all look good, there will only be ONE correct answer. You can do this! Just imagine you are in the clinical setting as you take this exam. The same type of reasoning you would use in clinical is necessary for NCLEX® SUCCESS!!!

1.5 ④ Option #4 is the correct answer. The client will need additional information since all of the motor function will not be regained. Support emotionally, spiritually, and psychologically will be of paramount importance for this client. Options #1, #2, and #3 are all correct statements and do not require additional information.

 I CAN HINT: A strategy to assist you in remembering the priority care for a client who has a diagnosis of a spinal cord injury is to remember "**PARALYZED.**"

Paralysis based on the location of the spinal cord injury

Assess urinary/bowel function

Respiratory depression/airway– acute; rehab– learn optimal level of independence

Assess neuro/LOC

Log roll; alignment is important

Yes circulation is important for perfusion

Zap out thrombus

Encourage protein/fluid

Derma tone/dermatology

1.6 ③ Option #3 is correct. High-risk behaviors, such as walking barefoot, using heating pads on the feet, wearing open-toed shoes, soaking the feet, and shaving calluses, should be avoided. Socks should be worn for warmth. Option #1 is incorrect. Feet should be examined each day for cuts, blisters, swelling, redness, tenderness, and abrasions. Option #2 is incorrect. Lotion should be applied to dry feet, but never between the toes. Option #4 is incorrect. After a bath, the client should gently, not vigorously, pat feet dry to avoid injury.

I CAN HINT: Safety is the key. With the risk of altered sensation for a client with Diabetes Mellitus, hot-water bottles and heating pads may burn the client. "CARE" will help you remember foot care for the client with diabetes.

Cut toe nails and foot care by podiatrist

Avoid hot-water bottles and heating pads

Review feet daily for redness, blisters, cuts, swelling, tenderness, and abrasions

Encourage patting feet dry after a bath to avoid injury to skin

1.7 ③ Option #3 is correct. The clinical presentation leads to a suspicion of abuse. It is important to get to the bottom line early in the assessment. Options #1 and #2 ignore the bruises. Option #2 focuses on the headache, which only had "some complaints," and the BP reading was not unusually high that would lead the nurse to be concerned with preeclampsia. Yes, the nurse does need to further assess the characteristics of the headache, but the immediate need is to determine the safety of this client. If the BP was elevated and/or the FHR was not a normal rate then there would be an immediate focus on the client's headache, VS, and FHR. This is not the current situation. Remember, the key is to make a clinical decision based on the information given in the stem of the question. Option #4 is vague and does not respond to the stem of the question.

 I CAN HINT: The key is to read the stem of the question carefully and answer what is being asked. The question is evaluating your ability to *"Assess client for potential or actual abuse."* The key assessments are *"bruises in various stages of healing on the abdomen and bilateral legs," "pregnant client and some complaints of headaches,"* and the *"VS and fetal heart rate."* There is not an indication of a complication with preeclampsia, such as hypertension, headache, etc. as outlined in the question. If there was a change in the BP and FHR and they were out of the normal range, then this would be an immediate physiological concern.

1.8 ② Option #2 is correct. This will assist client with establishing some control over behavior with no outside stimuli and activities for distraction. Option #1 would only contribute to the manic episode and would not be therapeutic. The last thing the nurse would want the client to engage in would be a competitive activity. Option #3 is incorrect. During the manic episode, the client is out of control and needs time to regroup. Option #4 is incorrect for the manic client. This would be appropriate if client was demonstrating manipulative behavior.

 I CAN HINT: "COMBAT" will assist you in organizing your care for a client who is becoming combative. An easy way to remember this is to think about time-out for a toddler who is acting out. The goal is to calm the client.

Control the immediate situation.

Out of situation (remove client by escorting to quiet room or a quiet location).

Maintain a calm behavior.

Be firm/set limits before becoming manic and combative.

Avoid restraints if possible.

Try consequences.

1.9 ③ Options #3 and #5 are correct. The key in
     ⑤ the stem of the question is "undiagnosed abdominal pain." The Do's for this diagnosis include: maintain on bed rest, place in a position of comfort, assess hydration, assess abdominal status: distention, bowel sounds, passage of stool or flatus, generalized or local pain, keep client NPO until notified otherwise. Option #1 is incorrect since the client should get nothing by mouth. Option #2 is incorrect. Do not apply heat to the abdomen. Cold applications may provide some relief or comfort. Option #4 is incorrect. Do not give narcotics for pain control before a diagnosis of appendicitis is confirmed, because this could mask signs if the appendix ruptures. The Do Not's for this diagnosis include: give nothing by mouth, do not put heat on the abdomen, no enemas, no strong narcotics, and no laxatives.

1.10 ① Option #1 is correct. This position will decrease the risk of reflux, which can lead to pulmonary damage if aspiration occurred. It is within the scope of practice for the UAP to position client in bed. Option #2 is not within the scope of practice for the UAP to assist with processing and reviewing plans for change based on client's concerns. Option #3 is incorrect. While it is appropriate for this client, it is not within the scope of practice of the UAP to review the reason, which is to prevent gastric dilation. Option #4 is incorrect. The use of pillows is not recommended as this can round the back, resulting in the stomach contents being closer to the chest.

 I CAN HINT: The key is, Standard of Practice + Scope of Practice = Successful answer! The majority of the time, a client with a gastric complication will have the HOB elevated to prevent aspiration.

1.11 ② The correct answer is option #2. Elderly adults may have difficulty swallowing. The HCP needs to be notified to change the order. Option #1 is incorrect. Some antibiotics cannot be given with milk and should not be crushed. The question was not specific enough to select this as an answer. Option #3 is incorrect since the elixir may require a dose change and this should be prescribed by the HCP, not the pharmacist. Option #4 is incorrect because this may result with the client choking.

1.12 ② Option #2 is the correct answer. Elevation of the HOB allows easier breathing. Option #1 is incorrect. Even if the client did require suctioning, the appropriate position would be to elevate the HOB versus to position them in the supine position. Option #3 is incorrect. There is no indication the client needs oxygen at this time. Even if the client did need oxygen, positioning would still be the priority for this question. Option #4 is incorrect for this question. While it may be important for the nurse to assess the lung sounds, it is not the priority for a client who is gasping in the middle of the night. Elevation of the HOB still remains the immediate priority.

1.13 ① Option #1 is the correct answer. Clients with diabetes mellitus have a problem with hyperglycemia. If a medication is ordered such as MethylPrednisolone Dose Pack that my elevate the blood sugar, then it is very important to monitor the serum glucose since the drug may work in opposition with the treatment for diabetes mellitus. Option #2 is incorrect. This does not answer the concern with the drug and disease. Option #3 is incorrect. While these packs may result in GI irritation, it is not addressing the question. Option #4 is incorrect. Vital signs are not answering the question.

1.14 ① Option #1 is the correct answer. A significant difference should be reported to the charge nurse. Option #2 is incorrect since there is an elevation in the blood pressure and it needs further evaluation. While option #3 is correct and needs to be documented, it is not a priority at this time. Option #4 would be note worthy, but not priority.

1.15 ④ Option #4 is the correct answer. Amlopdipine (Norvasc) is a calcium channel blocker. It blocks calcium access to the cells causing a decrease in contractility, thus resulting in a decrease in the blood pressure. Option #1 is incorrect since it has no action on the respiratory rate. Options #2 and #3 are incorrect for this drug category.

1.16 ② Option #2 is correct answer. This client mandates immediate assessment since there may be a need to initiate CPR if there is no pulse or respirations. Options #1, #3, #4 are not a priority over option #2.

1.17 ③ Option #3 is the correct answer. These clinical findings definitely indicate a complication with hypoglycemia. (Remember: *"Hot and dry blood sugar is high, cold and clammy means you need some candy!"*) It is imperative that client receives the milk to assist with the complication of hypoglycemia. Option #1 is incorrect. This does not address the complication presented by the client. Option #2 is incorrect. Insulin would further drive the blood sugar down. This would be inappropriate nursing care and would indicate a lack of understanding regarding the Standard of Practice for clients with hypoglycemia. Option #4 is incorrect. Intervention is a priority to increase the blood sugar prior to this action of notifying the HCP.

1.18 ④ Option #4 is correct. These 2 drugs may have an interaction that results in bleeding. Other drugs that may interact with warfarin (Coumadin) and result in bleeding may also include: garlic, ginger, ginseng, chamomile, etc. Option #1 is incorrect. Even though #1 may be attractive, this is not a nursing responsibility! Option #2 may be an accurate statement, but does not address the question regarding the client taking warfarin (Coumadin). Option #3 is also important, but not a priority over #4.

1.19 ② Option #2 is the correct answer. This drug is excreted by the kidneys and may result in nephrotoxicity if there is any complications with the renal system. The BUN and creatinine should be assessed prior to initiating this order and continue to monitor while taking the medication. Option #1 is an incorrect statement. Option #3 is incorrect. Option #3 is an appropriate nursing action due to the infection, but is not a priority over #2.

1.20 ④ Option #4 is the correct answer. It provides a legal explanation as to why the nurse is unable to respond to the mother's request. Option #1 is incorrect. Since the client is 21-years-old, the HCP is not legally able to provide information to the mother without the son's consent. Option #2 is avoiding responsibility. Option #3 is an accurate statement, but is a more adversarial statement than option #4.

1.21 ① ② ③ ④ Options #1, #2, #3, #4, are correct for this procedure. Option #5 is incorrect since sterile gloves and bandaging were used.

1.22 ④ Option #4 is most appropriate and reliable. Other acceptable ways to identify the client who does not have on an arm band may include: driver's license or a picture ID, phone number recall (if client alert), or have a client repeat and state name if client is alert and oriented and is not a very young child. Since this client is delusional, it is imperative to have a safe strategy for client identification. Stating name in this situation would not be appropriate. Options #1, #2 and #3 may not be reliable for this client who is elderly and delusional.

1.23 ② Option #2 is correct answer. Contact isolation is the appropriate isolation protocol for clients with Clostridium Difficile. Option #1 is incorrect. This is not a sporicidal and should not be used when coming in contact with client with Clostridium Difficile. Option #3 is incorrect. These clients should NEVER be in the same room. Option #4 is incorrect. Mask is not part of contact precautions unless the client is going to be suctioned or handling blood that is spurting, etc. The nurse should wear gloves and gown with this client and if the gloves are soiled during care, then these must be changed immediately.

1.24 ② Option #2 is the correct answer. An intramuscular injection requires a 1-1½ inch needle. The Bicillin is thick and will not easily go through the 25 gauge. Option #1 is incorrect because the needle is too long. Options #3 and #4 are incorrect because the gauge of the needle is too small.

1.25 ① Options #1, #2, #3, #5 are correct options
② for this pregnant client. Option #4,
③ turning the client to the left side and
⑤ providing only a small amount of oxygen are unlikely to assist with this emergency situation.

1.26 ① Options #1, #3, and #5 are correct
③ options. Option #2 may be comforting,
⑤ but also may make client feel there is an expectation that client will fall. Option #4 is likely to cause accidents.

1.27 ① Option #1 is always a priority for clients experiencing a seizure. Option #2 is not a priority over airway patency. Option #3 is not appropriate for this condition. Option #4 is important to implement to assist the client from falling, but if there is any

airway patency issue this will mandate intervention. The nurse will not just wait until seizure is finished if client is experiencing an obstructed airway.

1.28 ① Options #1, #2, #3, #4 are correct.
② Option #5 is incorrect since a full
③ assessment must be made prior to
④ reporting to the police.

1.29 Answer: 0.4mL. Available is 5 mg/mL and order is to administer 2mg. 5 mg in 1 mL, so 2 mg = 0.4 mL. Problem set up is: 5:1 = 2: X. Then cross multiply. 5X = 2. To solve for X divide each side of the equation by 5:

$$\frac{5X}{5} = \frac{2}{5}$$
$$X = 0.4$$

1.30 ② Option #2 is the correct answer. It is important to avoid sudden movement of the head and to avoid unnecessary nursing procedures. Room should be dimly lit and quiet. Option #1 is incorrect. The diet should be a low-sodium or low-salt diet. Option #3 is incorrect since the room should be quiet with minimal stimulation. Option #4 is incorrect since client should be on bed rest during an acute episode due to safety reasons. Client would be high risk for falling.

1.31 ③ Option #3 is the correct answer. Option #1 is incorrect since the specimen should not be collected from the drain. Option #2 is incorrect since the time of day is not relevant for a culture and sensitivity. Option #4 is not necessary for this procedure.

1.32 ③ Option #3 is the correct procedure. All other options are inappropriate for a child of this age. Injections should be administered in the vastus lateralis until the gluteus maximus is well developed, and this typically occurs after the child has been walking for 1 year.

1.33 Answer: 125 mL/hour. The nurse would divide the amount of fluid – 1000 mL by the number of hours—8—which is the infusion time for the IV fluid. 1000/8 = 125 mL/hour. Pumps are set at the rate per hour to infuse.

1.34 ②   Option #2 is correct. Clean gloves should be worn at all times when handling any client's body/body fluids. Option #1 is incorrect because it is only secondary to wearing a pair of clean gloves. Option #3 is incorrect because it may take a longer time to stop bleeding due to possibility of coagulation being altered due to impaired liver. Option #4 is incorrect because needles should never be recapped due to safety and risk of unnecessary needle sticks.

1.35 ③   Correct order is: 3, 1, 4, 2 ,5 , 6.
①
④
②
⑤
⑥

1.36 ④   Option #4 is the correct answer. Mild to moderate rashes are the most common side effects of Bactrim. Options #1, #2, #3 are not side effects of Bactrim.

1.37 ④   Option #4 is correct. This will increase the circulation and will decrease the risk of developing thrombophlebitis. Option #1 is incorrect because this will increase the risk by allowing blood to pool behind knee resulting in an increase risk for the development of thrombophlebitis. Option #2 is inappropriate. Option #3 is incorrect. It would be important to implement these actions while on bedrest; however, this answer does not address the question regarding the thrombophlebitis. It addresses potential pulmonary complications.

1.38 ③   Option #3 is correct. The Muslim culture believes that the same sex should provide care after death. Option #1 is incorrect since the Muslim culture grieves at home. Option #2 is inappropriate. Option #4 is incorrect since cremation is not practiced in the Muslim culture.

1.39 ②   Option #2 is correct. The therapeutic level for digoxin is 0.5-2.0 ng/mL. This level is toxic 2.2 ng / mL. The medication should be held. Option #1 is incorrect since it should not be given with this level. Option

#3 is an incorrect nursing action for this client. Option #4 is incorrect since the blood level of digoxin is the priority.

1.40 ②   Option #2 is correct due to safety issues. Options #1, #3, #4 are not going to hurt anyone.

1.41 ④   Option #4 is correct answer. The nurse should stand in front of the hearing impaired client. Option #1 is inappropriate for this situation because it is assuming the hearing loss is secondary to a build-up of wax. Option #2 is inappropriate for this situation. A sensory impaired client should always be aware that someone is present before being touched. Option #3 does not answer the question.

1.42 ②   Option #2 is correct. This is a priority when establishing a bladder or bowel retraining program. Option #1 is not correct since the schedule should be consistent and on a routine schedule versus a flexible schedule. While options #3 and #4 are part of the program, they are not a priority over option #2.

1.43 ①   Option #1 is the correct procedure. Options #2, #3,#4 are not accurate procedures for collecting a throat culture.

1.44 ①   Option #1 is the correct answer. Daily weights are the most appropriate and most measurable in determining the client's state of hydration. While options #2, #3, #4 are included in the assessment for evaluating hydration, they are not as measurable and objective regarding client's hydration as the daily weight.

1.45 ④   Option #4 is correct since nitroglycerin (Nitrostat) can cause hypotension. Clients should avoid changing positions quickly to decrease the risk of falling. Option #1 is incorrect. The nitroglycerin (Nitrostat) should be taken with the onset of pain. Option #2 is incorrect. A burning sensation or stinging sensation indicates the medication is working. Option #3 is incorrect. Nitroglycerin (Nitrostat) is sublingual and should not be swallowed.

1.46 ② Option #2 is correct. Option #2 is a priority with medication administration down the nasogastric tube. Verification of tube placement prevents the instillation of medications into the lungs which may result in aspiration pneumonia. While options #1, #3, #4 may be appropriate nursing interventions, they are not specific to the question regarding the priority nursing action prior to administering meds through a nasogastric tube and are not a priority over option #2.

1.47 ② Option #2 is correct. Sinequan is an antidepressant and signs of overdose include excitability and tremors. The other signs indicate depression which is the reason client is receiving this medication. Options #1, #3, #4 are not signs of Sinequan overdose.

1.48 ② Option #2 is correct. It is a convenient method for administering medications to an infant. Options #1 and #3 are incorrect. Infant may not take all of formula, so is usually not added to the bottle. Option #4 is incorrect due to the position of the infant. The supine position may increase risk for aspiration.

1.49 ④ Option #4 is an undesirable effect from furosemide (Lasix). All other options are desired outcomes of the drug.

1.50 ② Option #2 is correct. The permit must be signed prior to receiving pre-op meds. Client is considered incapacitated after receiving narcotics. Options #1, #3, #4 are incorrect.

1.51 ② Option #2 is correct. If the pulse rate drops below the set rate on the pacemaker, then the pacer is malfunctioning. The pulse should be maintained at a minimal rate set on the pacemaker. Options #1 and #3 do not indicate malfunction of the pacemaker. Option #4 may be an early sign of infection at site, but does not indicate a pacemaker dysfunction.

1.52 ① Option #1 is correct. Hypovolemia from bleeding is most likely the cause of the symptoms and should be assessed prior to contacting the healthcare provider. Option #2 is controversial, and is not a priority over bleeding assessment. Option #3 should have some additional assessments prior to contacting the healthcare provider. Option #4 is incorrect since pain is an unlikely cause of the symptoms of shock.

1.53 ④ Option #4 is correct. This assessment is evaluating the spinal accessory nerve (number 11). All other options are for different cranial nerves. Option #1 would be evaluating the hypoglossal nerve (number 12). Option #2 would be evaluating the first cranial nerve which is the olfactory nerve. Option #3 would be evaluating the 2nd cranial nerve which is the optic nerve.

1.54 ① ② ③ ④ Options #1, #2, #3, #4 are correct. The assessment did not indicate a broken area of skin and does not need to be isolated as indicated in Option #5.

1.55 ① Option #1 is the best option provided. This situation provides a legal dilemma and should be addressed immediately. Options #2, #3, #4 are inappropriate for this situation.

1.56 Answer: 25 gtts / minute. The nurse should divide 150 mL / hour by 60 minutes to get 2.5 mL / minute. Then multiply 2.5 mL / minute by 10 gtts / mL to get 25 gtts / minute at the rate to set the infusion set.

1.57 ③ Option #3 is the correct answer. This client is elderly; however, there is no indication that mobility is impaired. The greatest concern in evacuation is to move the largest number of clients initially, so those who are least critical are evacuated first. Option #1 is a client that has undergone major surgery, and is likely to be unable to ambulate due to anesthesia, and have an IV line in place. Option #2 is a client who is 6 hours post-op following an appendectomy.

Option #4 is a client that would also have an IV line in place, and would not be able to ambulate independently.

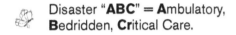 Disaster "**ABC**" = **A**mbulatory, **B**edridden, **Cr**itical Care.

1.58 ② Option #2 is correct. Aspirating the syringe with a subcutaneous heparin solution can cause bruising. Option #1 is incorrect. When administering Heparin, the site should not be massaged after administration. Options #3 and #4 are incorrect. Heparin is usually administered subcutaneously with a 5/8 inch needle into the abdomen.

1.59 ②
④
③
① The correct sequence for donning PPE is options #2, #4, #3, #1.

1.60 ② Option #2 is the correct option. Oxygen is highly flammable and clients who have oxygen in the home are at risk for a fire if an open flame is present. Options #1 and #3 are incorrect. Option #4 is a normal finding for a client with COPD.

NOTES

CHAPTER 2

Safe and Effective Care Environment:

Coordinated Care

*A genuine leader is not a searcher for consensus
but a molder of consensus.*
—Martin Luther King, Jr.

✔ Clarification of this test ...

The minimum standards include providing and directing activities that manage client care such as: client rights, confidentiality, information security, establishing priorities, managing staff conflict, client advocacy, collaboration with interdisciplinary team, quality improvement, referrals, informed consent, staff education and supervision.

- ☛ Provide information about advance directives
- ☛ Advocate for client self-advocacy
- ☛ Assign client care and/or related tasks (i.e., assistive personnel or LPN/VN)
- ☛ Involve client in decision-making about his/her care
- ☛ Contribute to the development and/or update of the client plan of care (i.e., client preferences, review current information)
- ☛ Participate as a member of an interdisciplinary team
- ☛ Recognize and report staff conflict
- ☛ Participate in staff education (i.e., in-services and continued competency)
- ☛ Use data from various sources in making clinical decisions
- ☛ Monitor activities of assistive personnel
- ☛ Maintain client confidentiality
- ☛ Provide for privacy needs
- ☛ Follow up with client after discharge
- ☛ Participate in client discharge or transfer
- ☛ Provide and receive report
- ☛ Organize and prioritize care for assigned group of clients
- ☛ Practice in a manner consistent with code of ethics for nurses
- ☛ Participate in client consent process
- ☛ Use information technology in client care
- ☛ Receive and process healthcare provider orders
- ☛ Recognize task/assignment you are not prepared to perform and seek assistance
- ☛ Respond to the unsafe practice of a healthcare provider (i.e., intervene or report)
- ☛ Follow regulation/policy for reporting specific issues (i.e., abuse, neglect, gunshot wound, or communicable disease)
- ☛ Provide care within the legal scope of practice
- ☛ Participate in quality improvement (QI) activity (i.e., collecting data or serving on QI committee)
- ☛ Apply evidence-based practice when providing care
- ☛ Participate in client data collection and referral
- ☛ Participate in providing cost-effective care

2.1 Which nursing action by the unlicensed assistive personnel (UAP) would require immediate intervention by the LPN for a client who had a cardiac catheterization 2 hours ago?

① Compare the quality of the pulses on the right and left legs.
② Evaluate the vital signs every 2 hours.
③ Encourage early ambulation to the bathroom to prevent a deep vein thrombosis.
④ Encourage oral intake of fluids following the procedure.

2.2 A client who is involved in a homosexual relationship is scheduled for abdominal surgery. During surgery, the partner requests information regarding her status. What is the appropriate response from the nurse?

① "The healthcare provider will be out to inform you after the surgery is complete."
② "HIPAA regulations and state laws will provide guidelines to assist with this decision."
③ "Let me go back and get an update. I will be right back with a report."
④ "She is doing fine; just sit back and relax."

2.3 Which of these nursing actions by the UAP for a client admitted to the cardiac unit with suspected heart failure would require intervention by the charge nurse due to the standard of care not being followed?

① Reports to the LPN that this client who is taking digoxin is complaining of nausea.
② Positions client in the low-Fowler's position with legs elevated.
③ Assists client to the bathroom due to frequent urination after receiving furosemide (Lasix).
④ Coordinates care with the LPN to provide uninterrupted sleep.

2.4 A client is scheduled to have a hip replacement and has signed the consent. What would be the priority of care if when completing the pre-procedure checklist the client says, "I don't really understand what they are planning to do! I don't think I want it done."

① Reassure the client that this is a routine surgery and there is nothing to worry about.
② Notify the surgeon that the client has questions and concerns about the procedure.
③ Answer the client's questions and explain the procedure.
④ Inform the client that the surgeon has already given consent for the surgery to be performed.

2.5 After receiving report on a surgical unit, which one of the following clients will you assess first?

① A 74-year-old male who had a hip replacement three days ago and is complaining of some mild pain.
② A 63-year-old female who is scheduled for an open reduction of her right wrist in the A.M. and has a temperature of 99.4°F.
③ A 78-year-old male who was admitted three hours ago after an open cholecystectomy and is complaining of the immediate need to urinate.
④ A 27-year-old female post-op hysterectomy admitted to the unit eight hours ago. Her significant other says she needs more pads because she is experiencing some small amounts of bleeding.

2.6 Which assignment would be appropriate to assign to the LPN / LVN?

① A 20-year-old client who has diabetes mellitus and is scheduled to be discharged today.
② A 50-year-old client with COPD who presents with distant breath sounds and needs an albuterol treatment.
③ A 30-year-old with bronchitis returning to floor after a bronchoscopy and needs initial assessment.
④ A 40-year-old client with a fractured femur in Russell's traction presenting with severe pain.

2.7 What room would be most appropriate to assign a client who has increased intracranial pressure following a head injury?

① The room closest to the nurses' station and elevator.
② The room with a room-mate who is active and very social.
③ A quiet room with no room-mates.
④ A room closest to lounge.

2.8 Prior to the physician inserting the chest tube, what nursing action would be most appropriate?

① Assess for allergies to penicillin.
② Assist client into the prone position.
③ Prep insertion site with soap and water.
④ Verify the consent form has been signed.

2.9 The LPN has assigned the task of obtaining vital signs to the UAP. The UAP reports to the LPN that one of the clients is requesting pain medication. What would be the most appropriate action for the LPN to make?

① Check the MAR to determine when the client was last medicated.
② Have the UAP repeat what the client said.
③ Assess the client.
④ Administer pain medication as ordered.

2.10 What is the priority of care for a client admitted with meningococcal meningitis?

① Administers morphine for complaints of headache.
② Wears gloves and gown when in contact with client.
③ Encourages frequent interaction to prevent sensory deprivation while hospitalized.
④ Reports the meningococcal infection to the health department.

2.11 The nurse receives a phone call to administer a preoperative sedative to a client who is scheduled to have surgery in the afternoon. When entering the room, the client states to the nurse, "I guess it is almost time for them to cut on me. Why can't they just give me medication to fix this?" What should the nurse do?

① Withhold the medication and notify the physician.

② Reassure the client that the surgery will go smoothly.
③ Administer the sedative to calm the client.
④ Review what the procedure will do for the client.

2.12 A 2-year-old is admitted to the hospital for dehydration secondary to severe diarrhea. The LPN is assigned to obtain a urine specimen from the child. What would be the best route for the nurse to take in order to obtain the specimen?

① Obtain an order for a straight catheter.
② Take the child to the bathroom and explain how to urinate in the specimen cup.
③ Explain the procedure to the parents and allow the parents to assist in obtaining the sample.
④ Tell the child they can have a piece of candy after they urinate in the specimen cup.

2.13 The LPN is assigned to care for a client with a history of frequent migraines, fibromyalgia, and irritable bowel syndrome. The client has received pain medication as ordered, but still reports a pain level 10/10 to the LPN. The LPN notifies the physician who states, "That client doesn't need more medication! They need a psychiatrist!" and angrily hangs up the phone. What should the LPN do next?

① Inform the client what the doctor said.
② Explain to the client why she may not have additional pain medication.
③ Obtain a referral for a psychiatrist.
④ Call the physician back and explain the assessment findings.

2.14 Which task can be delegated to the UAP for a client who has a nasogastric tube?

① Check the patency of the tube prior to taking client to bathroom.
② Disconnect the suction to allow ambulation to the toilet.
③ Remove the NG tube per provider of care's order.
④ Reconnect the suction after client has ambulated.

2.15 A client is admitted to the hospital for a therapeutic abortion. The LPN assigned to care for the client has a personal belief that abortion is wrong. The LPN informs the charge nurse that she does not want to care for the client due to personal beliefs regarding abortion. He/she is informed there are no other nurses available, and the assignment will not be changed. What is the next course of action for the LPN?

① Protest to the charge nurse again.
② Refuse to care for the client.
③ Provide prudent care to the client.
④ Notify the physician.

2.16 Which of these would be the most appropriate to assign to the LPN? *Select all that apply*. A client who:

① has the diagnosis of myasthenia gravis.
② is receiving chemotherapy.
③ is a new admission with chest pain.
④ is being discharged and needs new diabetic teaching.
⑤ is in Buck's traction.

2.17 Which of these situations does the LPN need to intervene with immediately? The UAP is:

① Giving a backrub to a client in traction.
② Taking routine vital signs.
③ Massaging the legs with lotion for a client with a deep vein thrombosis.
④ Straining the urine for a client with a kidney stone.

2.18 A wife is visiting her husband who has terminal lung cancer, COPD, and emphysema. The client has a signed living will that clearly states "Do not resuscitate." The client develops severe respiratory distress and the spouse runs into the hall screaming, "Someone do something! He is dying!" What should the LPN do?

① Comfort the wife, and encourage her to express her feelings of loss.
② Reinforce to the spouse that the client has a living will, and does not want CPR.
③ Assess the client, and administer prn xanax and albuterol.
④ Escort the wife back to the client's room, and then notify the family of the situation.

2.19 Which can be delegated to an experienced UAP?

① A 12-hour dietary recall from a client with bulimia.
② A urine specimen for a client with a UTI.
③ Document drainage from the pleur-evac.
④ Evaluate self-administration of insulin.

2.20 Which of these clients should be assessed first after receiving report? A client who is:

① Post bronchoscopy with HR–89 BPM, RR–22/min.
② Post op and received ½ unit of blood transfusion.
③ Complaining of pain following a liver biopsy.
④ Post-op with a HR–110 BPM, BP–98/62, IV infiltrated.

2.21 Which client should the LPN/LVN assess initially after shift report?

① A 30-year-old client who is complaining of itching on legs with diagnosis of Hepatitis A.
② A 40-year-old client who is complaining of epigastric pain during the night with a diagnosis of a duodenal ulcer.
③ A 50-year-old client presenting with chills who is scheduled for cardiac surgery in one hour. `
④ A 60-year-old client presenting with discomfort around the liver biopsy site.

2.22 Which of these clients should be evaluated immediately after report? A client:

① Post-bronchoscopy with a sore throat.
② Two hours after a gunshot wound with 1.0 cm of serosanguinous drainage.
③ Post-thyroidectomy with HR–88 BPM, RR–20/min., BP–120/80.
④ Post-tonsillectomy who is swallowing frequently.

2.23 During the night shift, an elderly client calls for the nurse. When the nurse enters the room, the client is sitting on the edge of the bed and states, "I fell in the bathroom, but I am okay." The nurse performs an assessment on the client and finds no apparent injury. What should the LPN do next?

① Make sure the light is on in the bathroom.
② Reevaluate the client every 30 minutes until morning.
③ Consult the agencies policy regarding falls.
④ Restrain the client for safety.

2.24 Which clinical assessment findings would be most important for the LPN/LVN to report for a 50-year-old client diagnosed with diverticulitis?

① HR–100, BP–102/68 from 140/78.
② Vague generalized abdominal discomfort.
③ Complaints of flatulence with abdominal tenderness.
④ Skin warm and dry with serum sodium of 144 mg/dL.

2.25 Which of these assignments should the LPN/LVN question?

① A client receiving routine antibiotic therapy for a wound infection.
② A client with diabetes mellitus who needs reinforcement in how to administer insulin.
③ A client newly admitted to begin chemotherapy.
④ A client admitted 3 days ago to the medical unit with asthma needing reinforcement with administering routine medications.

2.26 Which client assignment should the LPN/LVN question?

① An 80-year-old hospitalized yesterday with meningitis.
② A 2-month-old preparing for discharge tomorrow.
③ A client being admitted from home for a possible appendicitis.
④ A client with a GI bleed receiving the last 15 minutes of a blood transfusion.

2.27 The LPN/LVN is reviewing the budget with the staff, including the decision to change staffing ratios to include the use of more UAPs than LPNs. The staff is expressing concern over proposed staffing changes. What response made by the LPN/LVN would help assist the staff understand the principles behind the proposed changes?

① "We have to remain in our budget, and all willing to accept change to assure the budget is maintained."
② "The client ratio is being changed to reflect the needs of the client population in relation to the level of skill of the provider."
③ "The budget is not something that we can control, and we must learn to work within these financial limits."
④ "I know change is hard, but, this is something that needs to be done."

2.28 What should be the first nursing action by the LPN/LVN for a client experiencing a cardiac arrest with a DNR (Do Not Resuscitate) order?

① Assess the airway and give a breath.
② Call a Code.
③ Start an IV.
④ Evaluate client for signs of death.

2.29 The LPN/LVN is in charge of making assignments for the upcoming shift. When the staff arrives, they complain that they have an entirely different assignment than the previous day. What should the LPN/LVN do?

① Ask what the assignment was yesterday, and change the assignment to match it a closely as possible.
② Explain that the entire team has a job to do, and changing client's should not change that
③ Inform the staff that the assignment has been made, and that would not change.
④ Let the staff make the assignment.

2.30 The newly hired nurse is having extreme difficulty performing assigned duties in a timely fashion. Other members of the staff approach the LPN manager and complain. How can the manager handle this situation in an effective manner?

① Decrease the duties assigned to the new nurse.
② Tell the staff to express their concerns to the new nurse directly.
③ Schedule a performance review meeting with the new nurse.
④ Inform the new nurse that the staff is dissatisfied with her performance.

2.31 The LPN manager of a long term care facility obtained cleansing hand foam dispensers for all the client rooms, and pocket size hand sanitizer for all the staff to carry. Next, the LPN arranged for an in-service review of universal precautions and other safety concerns. What is the goal of these interventions?

① To comply with national standards of long term care facilities.
② To aid in managing cost effectiveness.
③ To instruct the staff on the personal benefits of using a hand sanitizer regularly.
④ To limit the use of soap and water to wash hands, as hand sanitizers are more effective.

2.32 The LPN at the long term care facility has noted that clients returning from physical therapy are in a lot of pain afterwards. Upon chart review, the nurse finds that many of the clients are not receiving medication prior to therapy. How can the nurse facilitate the need for clients to receive pain medication prior to therapy?

① Ask the therapy department for a schedule of therapy daily.
② Have the physician change the medication order from prn to a timed dosing.
③ Educate the client on the need for pain control.
④ Educate the staff on the requirement to medicate clients for pain after therapy.

2.33 Which of these phone calls should the LPN return first when working in an outpatient clinic?

① A pregnant woman in the last trimester who is complaining of insomnia when lying flat in bed.
② A client who is receiving chemotherapy and is complaining of nausea and anorexia.
③ A client with a cast on the left arm and is complaining of tingling in the fingers on the left hand.
④ A new mom who delivered 1 week ago and is complaining of discomfort when breastfeeding.

2.34 The LPN has arrived for the night shift. After receiving report on the assigned clients, which client should the nurse assess first?

① A 27-year-old who is requesting pain medication after undergoing an appendectomy 5 hours ago.
② A 55-year-old with diabetes and a blood sugar of 213 mg/dL.
③ A 60-year-old admitted with COPD who is requesting Xanax.
④ A 90-year-old admitted with a fractured hip following a fall.

2.35 Which of these assignments would be most appropriate to delegate to the pregnant LPN/ LVN?

① A client with a cervical radium implant.
② A client with syphilis.
③ A client with HIV.
④ A client with cytomegalovirus (CMV).

ANSWERS & RATIONALES

2.1 ③ The correct answer is option #3. The client should maintain bed rest; avoid flexion; keep extremity straight for 3 to 6 hours following the procedure. The UAP needs direction from the LPN regarding the standard of care for the client. This is dangerous to have the client up to the bathroom. Options #1, #2, and #4 are within the standard of care for this procedure. There is no need to immediately intervene with these nursing actions.

 I CAN HINT: The NCLEX® activity that you are being evaluated on here is "Use precautions to prevent injury and/or complications associated with a procedure or diagnosis." The key to answering this appropriately is to have an understanding of the care following the test. Let's use the mnemonic "**ACT NOW**" and see how this will work! I will not include the pretest preparation here such as NPO for 6 hours, assess allergies to iodine and contrast media, etc. We will focus on the **post procedure**.

Assess if the client is experiencing any allergies from the procedure

Check circulation (5 Ps: pulse, pain, pallor, paralysis, paresthesia—distal to cath site)

The provider of care should be notified for excessive bleeding at the site, changes in BP, or decrease in peripheral circulation or neurovascular changes in affected extremity. Teach as nursing care is being provided! It is an ongoing process!

Now NPO is over and client needs to be encouraged to drink fluids, IV access may be maintained

p**O**sition client with head of bed elevated at 30° or less; maintain bed rest; avoid flexion; keep extremity straight for 3 to 6 hours.

Watch for dysrhythmias, circulatory status changes, bleeding at site, vital sign changes drop in BP

We recommend you use this structure with each of your procedures as you study and review, so you will be ready for this part of the exam. STRUCTURE for organizing your thoughts and facts is the key to SUCCESS!!

2.2 ② Option #2 is the correct answer. Due to the HIPPA regulations and individual state laws, not all partners are recognized as legal partners. Since the NCLEX® is a national exam, the answers must represent all states. Option #1 is nurse avoidance. Option #3 violates HIPAA regulations. Option #4 is providing false reassurance and is not therapeutic.

 I CAN HINT: An understanding of HIPAA guidelines are important for answering this question accurately. "**HIPAA**," the privacy act, will include the following:

How to release information to healthcare providers that "need to know"

Impermissible uses and disclosures result in lawsuits

Protect privacy of individually identifiable health information

Arrange for sharing information with families in a discreet manner

Access by clients to medical records including the right to see and copy

2.3 ③ Option #2 is the correct answer. This nursing action is incorrect for this client. The client should be almost upright in bed with the feet and legs on the mattress in order to decrease venous return to the heart, which will result in a decrease cardiac workload. The elevation of the legs will increase the venous return causing an increase in the preload. This could be unsafe for this client due to the suspicion of heart failure. Options #1, #3, and #4 are all within the standards of care for a client with heart failure.

I CAN HINT: When answering the question, the key was to understand the care for a client with heart failure. In addition to the position of the client, it is important to consider other interventions for this client. "PERFUSE" will assist you in organizing this information.

Perfusion–peripheral, cerebral, renal

Evaluate vital signs, O₂ sat

Respirations characteristics (grunting, flaring, retracting)

Fluid status–weight, edema, heart/lung sounds

Use oxygen supplement safely

Stress–consolidate care, positioning, attention to T ↑, infections, anything that ↑ effort and ↑ calorie use

Evaluate activity tolerance

2.4 ② Option #2 is correct. It is the physician's responsibility to explain the procedure and to obtain the consent. The nurse can answer client's questions but it is ultimately the surgeon's responsibility. Option #1 is minimizing the client's concerns, and Options #3 and #4 are incorrect. Consent can always be withdrawn.

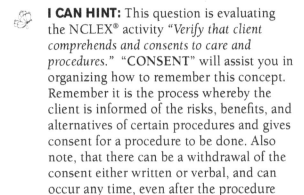 **I CAN HINT:** This question is evaluating the NCLEX® activity *"Verify that client comprehends and consents to care and procedures."* "CONSENT" will assist you in organizing how to remember this concept. Remember it is the process whereby the client is informed of the risks, benefits, and alternatives of certain procedures and gives consent for a procedure to be done. Also note, that there can be a withdrawal of the consent either written or verbal, and can occur any time, even after the procedure has begun.

Client competency is why nurse witnesses signature, validate the signature, ensure consent is voluntary.

Omit witnessing if client does not have all of the information to make an informed decision.

Note client understands the benefits and risks of the procedure.

Signed while client is free from mind-altering drugs or conditions; consent is a legal document.

Educated on alternatives to procedure; **E**mancipated minor: Definition may vary, but usually this is a minor who is self-supporting and living away from home.

Notes the healthcare provider performing the procedure.

Taught procedure to the client in terms she/he can understand

Exceptions for client to sign:

Life-threatening emergencies or urgent situations

Individuals are mentally incapacitated; Consent required of legal guardian or person specified to be medical of attorney.

For clients up to age 18, a parent's signature is generally required for consent.

2.5 ③ Option #3 is correct. If this client does not receive assistance, he may attempt to get up and could fall. This is a safety issue! The key word is "immediate." Option #4 is the second priority to assess for post-op bleeding. Option #1 is next to get pain medication. Option #2 has a low-grade temp, which will require notification of the provider of care, but is not a top priority.

I CAN HINT: The key is to understand how to prioritize. Since this requires higher level decision making, it will be imperative to make the decision based upon who you are "comparing and contrasting" with the options. A way to organize this would be around "**FIRST**." Please note that these are NOT in chronological order. They are several of the key concepts involved in prioritizing of care.

Find hypoxia (ABCs), fluid and electrolytes

Immunocompromised; increased intracranial pressure

Real bleeding! (significant increase in HR, drop in BP, etc.); rhythm changes with heart. Option #4: "A 27-year-old female post-op hysterectomy admitted to the unit *8 hours ago.* Her significant other says she needs more pads because she is experiencing some *small amounts of bleeding.*" is not a priority due to time and small versus significant amounts of bleeding.

Safety with risk for falls (Maslow). Option #3: "3 hours ago after an open cholecystectomy and is complaining of the *immediate need to urinate.*" is PRIORITY due to risk for falls when compared to other options.

Temperature and the complications

associated with procedures, surgeries, and medical conditions (i.e., pain, neurovascular changes, etc.); also need to review time frame that is given in question's stem and/or options. Option #1: "*3 days ago* and is complaining of some *mild pain*" is not a priority due to and characteristic of pain. Option #2: "open reduction of her right wrist in the A.M., and has a temperature of 99.4 degrees" is not a priority due to time for surgery and other client in option #3 has an immediate need.

2.6 ② Option #2 is the correct answer. This client is chronic, but does not require any initial assessment or teaching and is not presenting with a problematic outcome. Option #1 is not correct since discharge care will include teaching, and the LPN does not do initial teaching. Option #3 is not correct due to the initial assessment. Option #4 is incorrect since the presentation includes severe pain. This is a potential risk and mandates further assessment which may require analysis of the clinical findings.

I CAN HINT: "PART" represents part of the care the LPN is NOT able to do in isolation of the RN. **P**lan in isolation of the RN. LPNs plan in collaboration with the RN. **A**ssess initially: The LPN may perform ongoing assessments, but the initial assessment. **R**eview—Evaluate nursing care in isolation of the RN. The LPN must collaborate with the RN during this process. **T**eaching initially— The LPN may be involved in reinforcing teaching, but not the initial teaching. (*Nursing Made Insanely Easy* by Manning and Rayfield)

2.7 ③ Option #3 is the correct answer. The key to answering this successfully is to understand the need to decrease the stimulation. This option will decrease the external stimuli in the environment. Options #1, #2, #4 are incorrect due to the stimuli.

I CAN HINT: Room assignments: **RISK=** **R**adiation, **I**nfection/isolation, **S**timuli, Safety/sex, **K**now growth and development. (*Nursing Made Insanely Easy* by Manning and Rayfield)

2.8 ② Option #4 is the correct answer Verifying the consent has been signed is important to implement prior to this invasive procedure. Option #1 is incorrect. Option #2 is incorrect due to the position. Option #3 is an untrue statement.

2.9 ③ Option #3 is the correct answer. The nurse can delegate duties to the UAP; however, the UAP cannot make clinical decisions. The UAP reported pain to the LPN. It is the responsibility of the LPN to assess the client, and develop a plan of action to treat the client's pain.

I CAN HINT: The UAP "CAN'T" do the following: **C**annot make clinical decisions, **A**nticipate clinical changes, **N**o invasive procedures, **T**each. (*Nursing Made Insanely Easy* by Manning and Rayfield)

2.10 ④ Option #4 is the correct answer. It is imperative that this be reported to the health department. Options # 1, #2, and #3 are incorrect. Medicating the headache with a narcotic would mask neurological changes. Option #2 represents incorrect isolation standards. Option #3 is incorrect because the management should be the opposite in that the environmental stimulation needs to be decreased.

2.11 ① Option #1 is the correct answer. Informed consent prior to an invasive procedure requires the physician (not the nurse) to explain the procedure, risks, benefits, alternatives, and other issues specific to the procedure. Based on this scenario, the client does not understand why surgery is the only option for treatment. The physician should be notified, and the sedative withheld until the physician speaks to the client. Option #2 gives false reassurance. Option #3 will sedate the client and prevent dialogue with the physician. Option #4 is the role of the physician.

2.12 ③ Option #3 is the correct answer. This child is 2 years of age. Involving the parents and having the parents assist in the child's care will diminish separation anxiety. Option #1 is not appropriate for this client. This could result in an infection and is not a necessary action for obtaining a urine specimen for this child. Although a toddler's wish is to be independent, it is unlikely they will be able to provide a urine sample. It would not be appropriate to bribe a child with candy or another reward.

 I CAN HINT: "PRAISE" Push Pull toys, Parallel play, Rituals and Routines, Autonomy/Accidents, Involve Parents, Separation anxiety, Elimination, Explore. (Reference: *Nursing Made Insanely Easy*, by Manning & Rayfield)

2.13 ④ Option #4 is the correct answer. The client is reporting pain at 10/10. Pain is subjective, and is at the level that clients report. The physician was inappropriate in the response to the nurse, and it would be inappropriate to discuss this with the client. The nurse at this point does not have an explanation to give to the client regarding refusal of additional pain medication. A psychiatric referral is not indicated. The LPN must be an advocate for the client and attempt to discuss the assessment with the physician.

2.14 ② Option #2 is correct because it is within the scope of practice for the UAP. Option #1 is the responsibility of the LPN. UAPs do NOT assess. Option #3 is the responsibility of the nurse. Option #4 is incorrect. There will need to be additional assessment when the suction is reconnected, so the nurse is responsible for this action.

2.15 ③ Option #3 is the correct answer. The nurse is obligated to provide the same standard of care to all clients regardless of personal beliefs. Option #1 will not resolve the situation. Option #2 is unethical. Option #4 will not help change the situation.

2.16 ① Options #1 and #5 are correct because
⑤ they require general nursing care that is congruent with the Nurse Practice Act. Option #2 would require IV management and specialized assessment skills. Option #3 would require initial assessment. LPNs can do ongoing assessments, but it is not in the scope of practice to complete the initial assessment. Option #4 is incorrect because it requires initial teaching. The LPN can

reinforce teaching, but it is currently not in the scope of practice to do the initial teaching.

 I CAN HINT: The LPN does not do this "PART" of the nursing care! Plan in isolation of the RN, Push IV medications, Assess initially, Analyze, Review–evaluate in isolation RN, Teach initially.

2.17 ③ Option #3 is the correct answer. This action could dislodge a blood clot and result in a pulmonary embolus. Options #1, #2, and #4 are appropriate, and do not require immediate intervention due to unsafe care.

2.18 ③ Option #3 is the correct answer. The client has a living will that expresses his wishes; however, the client has not gone into cardiac arrest. It would be appropriate to assess the situation, and intervene to assist the client's current respiratory status. Option #1 is incorrect; the client has not expired. Option #2 ignores the client's condition. Option #4 is inappropriate.

2.19 ② Option #2 is the correct answer. This option involves a standard that involves a procedure that is unchanging. Option #1 cannot be delegated since it expects the UAP to evaluate the client which is not appropriate for the UAP. Option #3 is incorrect since it also involves evaluation. Option #4 is incorrect since the option evaluates a procedure, and is out of the scope of practice for the UAP.

2.20 ④ Option #4 is correct. This option indicates a complication with hypovolemia and needs IV fluid. The heart rate is rapid and blood pressure is low. Option #1 may be expected assessment findings. Option #2 does not indicate any complications with the blood transfusion. If there was a febrile reaction, then the option would have included assessments such as fever, chills, nausea, headache, flushing, tachycardia, palpitations. If the client was experiencing a hemolytic reaction, then assessment findings would be tachycardia, nausea, vomiting, decreased urine output, flushed face, burning at site, fever, chills, chest pain, hypotension, back pain. If client was experiencing an anaphylactic reaction, the assessment findings would include hives, itching, wheezing, stridor, pulmonary edema, flushed face, urticaria, general discomfort, increased temperature, chills/ chest pain, asthma, tachycardia. Option # 3 is an expected finding after this procedure.

2.21 ③ Option #3 is correct. Chills may indicate an infection, and the client needs further assessment immediately in order to determine if client has a temperature. Provider of care may need to cancel surgery due to an infection, but needs more clinical data to facilitate decision. While option #1 is a concern due to the pruritus, since this may be a result of jaundice and hyperbilirubinemia from the hepatitis, this is an expected physiological change and does not mandate an initial assessment after report in comparison to option #4. Option #2 is a concern, but does not mandate initial assessment, since this is an expected symptom with this condition due to the reduced gastric resistance to acid digestion. This would become a priority if the epigastric pain progressed to symptoms of hemorrhage, peritonitis, obstruction, etc. Option #4 is not a priority, since this is an expected outcome following this procedure. It would become a priority if the client was also presenting with hemorrhaging.

2.22 ④ Option #4 is correct. This client is hemorrhaging and requires immediate attention. Option #1 is an expected finding for this procedure. Option #2 is not a priority over a client who is actively bleeding. Option #3 is stable.

2.23 ③ Option #3 is the correct answer. Although the client is unharmed, the nurse is legally responsible to follow through with the agency's procedure regarding falls, and implement the policy exactly as written. Option #1 assumes the client has an issue with vision. Option #2 may be necessary, but without consulting the policy, the nurse would not know how often to assess the client. Option #4 is inappropriate. There is no indication the client is confused and in need of restraints.

I CAN HINT: LEGAL ASPECTS: due process, decision arbitrary, deprivation of property, deprivation of confidentiality

2.24 ① Option #1 is the correct answer. The client had a significant drop in the BP and HR – is 100. The client needs to be further assessed for bleeding. Options # 2 and #3 are not a priority over #1. Option #4 has a normal serum sodium level.

2.25 ③ Option #3 is the correct answer. A client receiving medication to treat cancer requires ongoing assessments from the RN. This client may experience unexpected outcomes. Options #1, #2, and #4 do not require an RN. There is no need to question these assignments.

I CAN HINT: PART: Plan, Assess, Review, Teach. The LPN can plan in collaboration with the RN, participate in ongoing assessments, collaborate evaluations, and reinforce teaching

2.26 ③ Option #3 is the correct answer. This client is being admitted to the hospital, and it is not in the scope of practice for an LPN/LVN to make an initial assessment. Options #1, #2, and #4 represent clients who are already in the healthcare system. It is appropriate for the LPN/LVN to provide care to these clients in collaboration with the registered nurse.

I CAN HINT: PART: Plan, Assess, Review, Teach. The LPN can plan in collaboration with the RN, participate in ongoing assessments, collaborate evaluations, and reinforce teaching.

2.27 ② Option #2 is the correct answer. Cost effectiveness must be a consideration in management. The changing of staff skill level to reflect the needs of the client is appropriate. If the client population does not require skilled care, it is appropriate to assign a nursing assistant vs. an LPN / LVN. Option #1 is not informative regarding the reason for the change. Options #3 and #4 do not identify the need (rationale) for the change. They just identify change must take place.

I CAN HINT: SAVE = Staff, Avoid duplication, View infection, Educate

2.28 ④ Option #4 is the correct answer. A written order is mandated for a DNR (Do Not Resuscitate). This requires no invasive or out of the ordinary care to be implemented such as CPR, medications, ventilation, etc. Options #1, #2, #3 are incorrect for this order.

2.29 ① Option #1 is the correct answer. When possible, it is beneficial to the client to have the same care providers because a relationship exists between the client and provider. Options #2 and #3 are inflexible and disregard the lack of continuity in client care. Option #4 is not appropriate. The LPN is assigned the charge nurse role and is responsible for the shift and the unit as a whole.

2.30 ③ Option #3 is the correct answer. The new nurse is learning, and it is important to identify areas that need to be improved upon, such as timeliness, and develop a plan to meet that goal. Option #1 is not correct. The new nurse needs to be able to perform assigned duties. Option #2 is not appropriate, as the new nurse is likely to feel "attacked" by the staff. Option #4 does not explore the issue, and will not promote team work.

2.31 ② Option #2 is the correct answer. Infections are detrimental to the client, and are expensive to treat. Providing equipment and reviewing standard (universal) precautions with the staff are a means to help prevent infections from occurring. Option #1 is not correct. Option #3 implies the benefits are on a personal level for the staff. Option #4 is incorrect. Soap and water hand washing are as effective as hand sanitizers. Hand sanitizers are an option, but do not replace soap and water.

I CAN HINT: SAVE = Staff, Avoid duplication, View infection, Educate

2.32 ① Option #1 is the correct answer. By asking the therapy department for a schedule, the nursing staff can offer pain medication to the client prior to therapy. This will help reduce discomfort to the client, increase compliance while in therapy, and improve the quality of care to the client. Option

#2 is not indicated. The pain medication is available, and round the clock pain medication is not appropriate for all clients. Option #3 does not help resolve the issue of timing pain medication for therapy clients. This option also implies the client is responsible for pain control. It is the responsibility of the nurse and the client. Option #4 states there is a requirement for medication, which is not appropriate for all clients. It would be more effective to manage pain prior to physical therapy if there is a prn medication ordered.

2.33 ③ Option #3 is the correct answer since this may indicate some neurovascular compromise mandating immediate attention to prevent further damage. Options #1, #2, and #4 are all expected outcomes for these clients. Option #1 needs to change positions when sleeping to either the left side or upright. Option #2 will be nauseated with minimal appetite when receiving chemotherapy. Option #4 will experience some discomfort due to the release of oxytocin when breastfeeding.

2.34 ③ Option #3 is the correct answer. The client with COPD is requesting Xanax which indicates the client is anxious. A common cause of anxiety in clients with COPD is shortness of breath. Options #1, #2, and #4 need attention from the nurse, but are not the priorities over #3.

 I CAN HINT: Prioritizing using the "FIRST" method:
Find hypoxia
Immunocompromised
Real bleeding
Safety
Try Infection

2.35 ③ Option #3 is the correct answer because an HIV client would not present a risk to the pregnant woman if she does not come in contact with the body secretions. Options #1, #2, #4 could result in teratogenic effects to the fetus.

CHAPTER 3

Safe and Effective Care Environment:

Safety and Infection Control

*You can't make positive choices for the rest of
your life without an environment that makes
those choices easy, natural, and enjoyable.*
—Deepak Chopra

✔ Clarification of this test ...

The minimum standards include performing and directing activities that manage client care
such as medical/surgical asepsis, standard/universal precautions, identification of allergies,
use of restraints, safe use of equipment, accident prevention, error prevention, handling
hazardous and infectious materials, incident reports, and safety precautions.

- ☞ Identify client allergies and intervene as appropriate
- ☞ Verify the identity of client
- ☞ Assist in or reinforce education to client about safety precautions
- ☞ Evaluate the appropriateness of healthcare provider order for client
- ☞ Participate in preparation for internal and external disasters (i.e., fire and natural disasters)
- ☞ Use safe client handling (i.e., body mechanics)
- ☞ Use transfer-assistive devices (i.e., gait/transfer belt, slide board, and mechanical lift)
- ☞ Identify and address hazardous conditions in healthcare environment (i.e., chemical, smoking, and biohazard)
- ☞ Acknowledge and document practice error (i.e., incident reports)
- ☞ Follow protocol for timed client monitoring (i.e., restraint, safety checks)
- ☞ Implement least restrictive restraints or seclusion
- ☞ Assure availability and safe functioning of client-care equipment
- ☞ Initiate and participate in security alert (i.e., infant abduction or flight risk)
- ☞ Identify the need for and implement appropriate isolation techniques
- ☞ Use standard/universal precautions
- ☞ Use aseptic and sterile techniques

3.1 Which nursing actions should a nurse implement for a client with tuberculosis? *Select all that apply.*

① Restrict visitors to immediate family only.
② Put on a gown.
③ Wear N95 respirator mask.
④ Place in a negative pressure room.
⑤ Wear gloves when in contact with the client.

3.2 A client on chemotherapy has a WBC count of 1,200/mm. Based on this data, what is the priority nursing action?

① Check temperature q 2-4h.
② Monitor urine output.
③ Assess for bleeding gums.
④ Obtain an order for blood cultures.

3.3 What instructions should the nurse reinforce in the discharge teaching for a client who was admitted to ER for a suspected outbreak of anthrax, that was transmitted by skin exposure, and who has received a prescription for antibiotics from the healthcare provider? *Select all that apply.*

① Wear a N95 mask for 45 days.
② Remain in respiratory isolation during the time on antibiotics.
③ A black eschar forms over the lesion and will dry and fall off in 1 to 2 weeks.
④ Antibiotics should be taken for a duration of 60 days.
⑤ The drainage from the lesions will be cloudy serous fluid.

3.4 What plans should be implemented for clients with sealed radioactive implants? *Select all that apply.*

① When close to client or prolonged care is required use a lead shield or wear a lead apron.
② Limit visitors to 60 minutes per day.
③ Advise visitors to stay about 6 feet from the client.
④ Keep long-handled forceps and lead container in room in case of dislodgment of a radioactive source.
⑤ Discard all dressings and bed linens as soon as removed from client.

3.5 Place in chronological order the sequence of events for the nurse to implement in a Code Red (fire alarm). **Use all of the options.**

① Contain the fire.
② Aim the extinguisher at the base of the fire.
③ Activate the alarm.
④ Pull the pin on the extinguisher.
⑤ Extinguish the fire from side to side.
⑥ Remove any clients from the fire.

3.6 The nurse is going to transfer a client using a hoyer lift. The nurse is aware that the most important assessment to make prior to transferring the client with the lift is:

① verify the client is ready to transfer.
② determine if help is available.
③ verify placement of the lift pad.
④ determine the lift is correctly functioning.

3.7 The nurse observes a UAP preparing to transfer a client from the bed to a wheelchair. The client has a history of right-sided weakness. Which observation made by the nurse requires immediate attention? The UAP:

① places the wheelchair parallel to the bed as close as possible to the bed.
② has applied a gait belt to the client.
③ has not applied both brakes.
④ has not enlisted assistance.

3.8 A client who has metastatic colon cancer is under the care of the LPN. The client states to the LPN, "I have decided to start smoking again. Could you get me a wheelchair, so I can go outside?" How should the LPN respond to the client's request?

① "I cannot allow you to leave the unit without notifying the physician."
② "Starting to smoke again is not a good choice for someone with your diagnosis."
③ "Do you have someone to accompany you outside?"
④ "Clients are not allowed to leave the unit to smoke."

3.9 A client in a long-term facility has a long history of Insulin Dependent Diabetes Mellitus (IDDM), and the nurse is reviewing the plan of care for the client. Which intervention, if ordered, should the LPN question?

① an 1800 calorie diabetic diet

② provide foot care every other day

③ finger stick blood sugars before meals and at bedtime

④ ambulate the client to the dining room for meals

3.10 Which of these nursing actions indicate the nurse understands how to safely provide care for a client with a Streptococcal (Group A) pharyngitis? The nurse wears:

① A gown when entering the room.

② Gloves when taking blood pressure.

③ A surgical mask when 5 feet from client.

④ Surgical mask when 2 feet from client.

3.11 Which of these medications should the nurse question?

① Digoxin for an adult client with a heart rate of 64.

② Enalapril (Vasotec) for a client being discharged post MI.

③ Hydrochlorothiazide (HCTZ) for a client with stage I hypertension.

④ Carvedilol (Coreg) for a client with COPD.

3.12 The LPN is caring for a client who had internal radioactive therapy. The client calls the nurse, and when the nurse enters the room the client points to one of the implants in the sheets. What intervention should the nurse do next?

① Don a lead apron and gloves prior to entering the room.

② Put on gloves, pick up the implant and place in a lead box.

③ Pick up the implant with long forceps and place in a lead box.

④ Have the client put the implant in a lead box.

3.13 The LPN is working for a home healthcare agency. Which finding, if observed, would be of greatest concern to the nurse?

① a client with an infected wound and allows cats to eat off the table

② a client receiving intermittent oxygen therapy and has a spouse that smokes in the home

③ a client with diabetes who has a bowl of candy sitting on the coffee table

④ a client with COPD sleeps in a recliner instead of a bed

3.14 The LPN is teaching a parenting class at the local community center. Which statement made by the parents indicates a need for further instruction?

① "I will keep medications, like aspirin, on hand in case my child becomes ill."

② "I will lock all the cleaning supplies in a cabinet."

③ "I will enroll in a refresher CPR class as soon as possible."

④ "I will make sure to cut up foods, like hot dogs, into small pieces."

3.15 Which action indicates a mother with Hepatitis A understands how to protect her family from the transmission of Hepatitis A?

① Mother refuses to hold newborn in order to prevent transmission of Hepatitis A.

② Mother eats meals in a different room from the rest of the family.

③ Mother refuses to let children to take drinks out of her glass.

④ Mother refuses assistance with child care.

3.16 Which information would be most important to instruct a client about who has Hepatitis B?

① Discuss the importance of eating a diet high in protein and low in carbohydrates for each of the three meals.
② Instruct client regarding the importance of continuing to having intimate relations with husband.
③ Review the importance of using own towels for shower.
④ Discuss the importance for client to wear a mask when in contact with others.

3.17 The nurse is aware that a priority consideration to take into account when preparing to perform a sterile dressing change is:

① the ability of the client to cooperate.
② the availability of assistance.
③ the client's understanding of the procedure.
④ the presence of visitors in the room.

3.18 An LPN working on a medical unit hears an overhead notification of a possible infant abduction. The nurse recognizes her primary response is:

① to monitor the exit doors.
② to detain anyone looking suspicious.
③ to lock all exits to the unit.
④ to notify security of anyone carrying a large bag.

3.19 A client is to be admitted with the diagnosis of hepatitis, pancreatitis, MRSA, hypertension, and alcoholism. To prepare the client's room, it is important for the nurse to obtain:

① padded side rails.
② bed side commode.
③ masks, gowns, gloves, and goggles.
④ telemetry monitor.

3.20 The LPN observes the UAP bending over at the waist when assisting a client to get out of bed. What is the priority nursing action?

① Do nothing since the UAP has the care under control.
② Discuss appropriate body mechanics with the UAP to prevent injury to self.
③ Assist the UAP in getting client out of bed.
④ Send UAP through a complete orientation program.

3.21 A client is agitated and combative. The nurse is aware that the situation needs to be resolved. Which intervention made by the nurse would be the least effective?

① removing client from the environment
② being firm with the client
③ removing harmful objects, such as silverware
④ detaining the client and applying restraints

3.22 A client in the community is contaminated from anthrax by an aerosolizable spore containing powder. Which of these nursing actions indicate the nurse understands how to safely manage client?

① Review the importance of post-exposure prophylaxis following exposure for 30 days with levofloxacin (Levaquin).
② Use standard precaution when working with the client.
③ Wash hands with alcohol hand rubs if become contaminated.
④ Wear respirator N95 mask and protective clothing until decontamination of environment is complete.

3.23 A 79-year-old client lives alone at home. Which question is the highest priority for the nurse to ask in regards to the client's safety?

① "Do you know what temperature you have your thermostat set?"
② "Do you have soft glow light bulbs in your room lamps?"
③ "Do any of your current medications cause you to feel unsteady or weak?"
④ "Have you considered selling your home and moving into an assisted living area?"

3.24 What is the best way to prevent accidents with equipment in the hospital?

① Always have a person to assist the nurse prior to using equipment.
② Always unplug the equipment when moving the client.
③ Always lock wheels on movable equipment.
④ Never operate equipment without previous education and instruction.

3.25 A client with Chronic Obstructive Pulmonary Disease was diagnosed with carbon dioxide retention and has a pulse oximetry reading of 80% on room air. The provider of care orders 40% Oxygen via mask. What would be the priority of care?

① Notify respiratory therapy to initiate the order.
② Assess breath sounds prior to administering the oxygen.
③ Notify the provider of care and verify the appropriateness of this order.
④ Provide meticulous care around face and nose due to potential skin breakdown.

3.26 A client comes in for treatment of pneumonia and a healthcare provider orders Cefazolin (Ancef). The nurse notes the client has a Penicillin allergy. What is the priority nursing intervention?

① Verify the order.
② Check the client's temperature.
③ Observe the client for rash or swelling.
④ Administer as ordered.

3.27 When doing a dressing change on a client with an abdominal wound, which nursing actions would be most appropriate? *Select all that apply.*

① Wash hands.
② Squeeze antibiotic ointment directly on the wound.
③ Pour antiseptic cleaning agent from an unsterile bottle after putting on sterile gloves.

④ Saturate cotton balls with the cleaning agent.
⑤ Work from the top of the incision, wiping once to the bottom and then discard the pad.
⑥ If client has a surgical drain, clean drain surface first.

3.28 To promote client safety, which pieces of equipment should be readily available at the bedside when client has a seizure disorder? *Select all that apply.*

① Oral airway
② Nasogastric tube
③ Suction
④ Ventilator
⑤ Tracheostomy set

3.29 To promote client safety, which nursing action would be a priority for the LPN to implement when assisting the RN to obtain a blood specimen from a client with hepatitis B?

① Cleanse area with antiseptic solution.
② Apply pressure to site for 5 seconds.
③ Recap needle to avoid carrying exposed needle.
④ Wear a pair of clean gloves.

3.30 Select the correct procedures when following standard (universal) precautions. *Select all that apply.*

① Wear a face shield when entering the room.
② Wear gloves when coming in contact with any body fluid.
③ Place the client in a private room that has negative air pressure in relation to surrounding area.
④ Discard used needles immediately in the trash can.
⑤ Wear gloves when entering the room.
⑥ Avoid contact with client if nurse has an exudative lesion.

3.31 Following hip replacement surgery, an elderly client is ordered to begin ambulation with a walker. In planning nursing care, which statement by the nurse will best help this client?

① "Sit in a low chair for ease in getting up to the walker."
② "Make sure rubber caps are present on all four legs of the walker."
③ "Begin weight-bearing on the affected hip as soon as possible."
④ "Practice tying your own shoes before using the walker."

3.32 Which of these nursing actions indicate an understanding of safe use of restraints?

① Remove or replace restraints every shift.
② Pad bony prominences and do neurosensory checks twice a shift.
③ Tie the restraint to the bed frame with loose knots.
④ Limit range of motion with the restraints and with enough room to fit 1 finger between the device and the client to prevent injury.

3.33 What is the priority plan for preventing falls in the older adult?

① Recommend removing all rugs in the home.
② Encourage installation of appropriate lighting in the home.
③ Review the normal aging changes that place one at risk.
④ Complete a comprehensive risk assessment.

3.34 Which of these home care instructions should the LPN reinforce to the parents of a child who had been exposed to human immunodeficiency virus (HIV)?

① Avoid all immunizations until diagnosis has been confirmed.
② Avoid sharing toothbrushes.
③ Wipe up spills of blood with soap and water.
④ Wash hands with ½ strength Bleach if comes in contact with child's blood.

3.35 What should be the priority of care for a client admitted with severe hypoparathyroidism?

① Provide extra blankets in the room.
② Keep room cool.
③ Initiate seizure precautions.
④ Lower the head of the bed.

ANSWERS & RATIONALES

3.1 ③ Options #3, #4, and #5 are correct.
④ Airborne precautions are used in addition
⑤ to standard precautions for clients who are known or suspected to be infected or colonized with infectious organisms. Diseases known to be transmitted by air for infectious agents smaller than 5 mcg (measles, varicella, pulmonary or laryngeal tuberculosis) must follow these precautions as outlined by CDC. PPE should include gloves, mask (N95 respirator) for known or suspected TB. In addition to standard precautions, the client should be in a monitored negative airflow (air exchange and air discharge through HEP filter). Doors of the room should be kept closed. If client leaves room, a small, particulate mask should be applied to the client if leaving room for medical necessity. Options #1 and #2 are not essential in airborne precautions.

3.2 ① Option #1 is correct. It is important to monitor for infection which would be evidenced by an elevated temperature in a client who has such a low WBC count. Option #2 is important to monitor because of problems of increased uric acid excretion from chemo-therapeutic drugs, but is not applicable to this situation. Option #3 would be associated with a low platelet count. Option #4 would be secondary to option #1, but currently there is not any clinical findings that mandate an order for a blood culture.

 I CAN HINT: The key here is to know the normal WBC count is 5,000–10,000/mm3 and the link to this lab value is a sign of infection. There must be a sign of infection prior to obtaining an order for blood cultures. The goal is to place these clients in protective environment precautions in order to prevent infections from occurring. The clients that typically require this type of isolation include clients who: (1) have an increased susceptibility to infections, (2) are receiving chemotherapy, or (3) are immuno-suppressed or neutropenic.

Minimize exposure to microorganisms found on the outer layers of fresh flowers, fruits, and vegetables. Follow the transmission precautions outlined by CDC when in contact with client. Maximum protection will require ventilated positive pressure room. In addition to these precautions, Standard Precautions should also be implemented.

3.3 ③ Options #3 and #4 are correct. Even if the
④ symptoms do not persist, the client must take the antibiotics for 60 days. A painless lesion will develop with a black eschar at the center. The lesion usually remains localized, though if untreated systemic infection may develop. Incubation periods range from 1 to 12 days. The lesion begins as a painless, pruritic macular or popular lesion, much like an insect bite. By day two the lesion has swollen, vesiculates, and ruptures to from depressed ulcer. Smaller lesions may form around the primary lesion. Option #5 is incorrect since the clear serosanguineous fluid in these lesions contains large quantities of bacilli. The area surrounding the lesion will be swollen. Option #3, the black eschar forms over the depression, dries, and falls off in 1 to 2 weeks. Lesions affecting the head and neck may have significant swelling. Options #1 and #2 are incorrect. There is no human-to-human infection.

I CAN HINT: The key to answering this question accurately is to understand the specific facts about anthrax. "**ANTHRAX**" will organize this for you.

Agent: Bacillus anthracis

No human-to-human infection

Treatment: antibiotic therapy for 60 days

Has an incubation period of 1 to 12 days

Reported cases: cutaneous anthrax accounts for 95%

Assessments: A painless lesion develops with a black eschar at the center;

X out (black eschar) will form over the depression, dry, and fall off in 1 to 2 weeks.

3.4 ① Options #1, #3, and #4 are correct. When
③ close to client or prolonged care is required
④ use a lead shield or wear a lead apron.
This is included in the standard of care for
sealed radioactive implants. Option #3 is
correct. Visitors should stay about 6 feet
from the client to promote safety. Option
#4 is correct. Keeping a long-handled
forceps and lead container in room in case
of dislodgment of a radioactive source are
included in the standard of care. Options
#2 is incorrect. The time frame should be
30 min. per day. Option #5 is incorrect. All
of the dressings and bed linens should be
saved until radioactive source is removed;
follow guidelines from radiation safety
officer.

 I CAN HINT: Safety precautions to prevent
excessive exposure for healthcare providers
are the key to answering the question
accurately. Remember *Distance*, *Time*, and
Shield will assist you in organizing the
nursing care.

Distance: maintain the maximum distance
possible to provide care. Attempt to
maintain distance of 6 feet from the
source of radiation.

Time: Coordinate care to minimize caregiver's exposure.

Shield: When close care or prolonged care
is required, use a lead shield or wear a
lead apron. Wear a film badge to measure
exposure; do not share film badges.

3.5 ⑥ Remove any clients from the fire.
③ Activate the alarm.
① Contain the fire.
④ Pull the pin on the extinguisher.
② Aim the extinguisher to the base of the fire.
④ Extinguish the fire from side to side.

 I CAN HINT: The strategies for answering
this question is to use the acronym
"RACE" to assist you in remembering the
emergency fire response. Fire extinguisher
safety can be recalled by another acronym:
"PASS"

Rescue	**P**ull the pin
Activate	**A**im at the base of the fire
Contain	**S**queeze the trigger
Extinguish	**S**weep from side to side

3.6 ④ Option #4 is correct. It is always a priority
to determine if the equipment is working
appropriately prior to using for client care.
Options #1, #2, and #3 are not a priority
over option #4 since this is about safety.

3.7 ③ Option #3 requires immediate attention
since this is a safety hazard for the client.
Option #1 should actually be placed on the
unaffected side, so the strong side will lead
in helping client get out of bed. Option #2
is not a safety issue. Option #4 may be a
concern, but definitely is not a priority over
option #3.

3.8 ② Option #2 is a truthful and informative
response to a client with this diagnosis.
Options #1, #3 and #4 are not providing
information to the client to assist with the
recovery.

3.9 ② Option #2 is the correct answer. Diabetics
are at high risk for injury/damage to
the lower extremities. It is essential that
diabetics are instructed to evaluate their
feet daily, wear closed toe shoes that fit
well with cotton socks, and report any
abnormalities immediately. This standard is
also appropriate for a client in a long term
care facility, and the nurse should evaluate
the client's feet daily. Options #1, #3, and
#4 are all appropriate interventions for the
diabetic client.

3.10 ④ Options #4 is the correct answer. The
infection control guidelines outline the
need to wear a mask when 3 feet from the
client with this infection. Option #1 is not
necessary for this client when entering the
room. If the client needed to be suctioned,
had blood spurting out, was incontinent
with diarrhea, or needed a wound irrigated,
then gown would be necessary. Option #2
is not necessary for this client. This would
be important if the client needed contact
isolation such as if they had MRSA, VRE, a
major abscess, or a decubitus. Option #3 is
incorrect for this client as outlined in first
part of rationale.

3.11 ④ Option #4 is the correct answer. It is a nonselective beta blocker and may result in bronchoconstriction. (Refer to *Pharmacology Made Insanely Easy*, by Manning, Loretta and Rayfield, Sylvia for memory technique.) Option #1 does not need questioned. This does not reflect bradycardia. Option #2 is appropriate for this client. Ace inhibitors are appropriate for clients after a myocardial infarction since these drugs suppress the rennin–angiotension-aldosterone system by blocking the conversion of angiotensin 1 to angiotensin 2 (a potent vasoconstrictor). This may result in a decrease in the systemic and peripheral vascular resistance and will decrease left ventricular dilation after an MI. Option #3 does not need to be questioned since this diuretic will be therapeutic for this client.

3.12 ③ Option #3 is the correct answer. The nurse should pick the implant up with long forceps and place in a lead box to avoid exposure. Option #1 is incorrect, it is not necessary to use this equipment for a radioactive implant, and does not answer the question since the nurse is already in the room. Option #2 is incorrect as gloves will not protect against the radioactive implant. Option #4 is incorrect. Appropriate containment of the radioactive agent is the duty of the nurse.

3.13 ② Option #2 is the correct answer. Oxygen is highly flammable and clients who have oxygen in the home should not smoke in the home. While options #1 and #3 may be a concern, they are not a priority over option #2. Option #4 is a normal finding in a client with COPD.

3.14 ① Option #1 is the correct answer. Although it is correct to keep medications on hand, aspirin is never an appropriate choice for children due to Reye's syndrome. Options #2, #3, and #4 are correct statements and do not mandate any further instruction.

3.15 ③ Option #3 is the correct answer. Hepatitis A can be transmitted by sharing eating utensils and / or drinking glasses. Hands should be washed before eating and after using toilet. High risk groups include children, international travelers, poor sanitation, no preparation of food, etc. Option #1 is incorrect. It is not transmitted by contact. Option #2 is incorrect. She can eat with family, but just not share her eating utensils. Option #4 is not correct since she should accept assistance due to needing time to heal.

3.16 ③ Option #3 is the correct answer. Hepatitis B is transmitted through blood and body fluids. Individuals who are high risk for this include: transfusions, individuals who use drugs, men who are homosexual, health-care workers, etc. Linens should never be shared with individuals who have Hepatitis B. Option #1 is incorrect. It is recommended that meals are small and frequent and they include high calories and carbohydrates. Option #2 is incorrect. Sexual contact should be avoided until serologic indicators have returned to normal. Option #4 is incorrect. This is transmitted by blood and body secretions. There is no rationale for wearing a mask since it is transmitted through blood and body secretions.

3.17 ① Option #1 is the correct answer. If a client is unable or unwilling to cooperate with a dressing change, it will be very challenging for the nurse to maintain sterile technique. For example, if a client is confused and the nurse is changing a wound on the abdomen, it will be difficult to keep the client from reaching at the nurse or wound. Option #2 would be appropriate, only if assistance is needed, which cannot be determined without determining the client's ability to cooperate. Option #3 is important to assess prior to beginning the procedure, but not a priority over option #1. Option #4, the presence of visitors would be a concern at the bedside, not in the preparation. Visitors can be asked to step out of the room when the nurse plans to perform a skill such as a sterile dressing change, or asked to move away to maintain the sterile field.

3.18 ① Option #1 is the correct answer. The role of the nurse is to monitor exits from the hospital. In an instance of infant abduction, the infant could be in a small bag, inside a shirt or another small item. It is imperative to not let anyone leave the building until the infant has been located. Option #2 is incorrect. The nurse cannot physically detain someone based on appearance, but can notify security of suspicions. Option #3 is incorrect. If there was an emergency, such as a code, the medical team must be able to access the unit. Option #4 is incorrect as an infant can be placed in a very small bag as previously discussed.

3.19 ③ Option #3 is the correct answer. All clients' care requires the use of standard (universal) precautions, but the diagnosis of MRSA requires the nurse to prepare for additional precautions. Although it is not identified where the MRSA is located, the nurse should be prepared to care for the client regardless of the location of the infection. Option #1 would be appropriate for a client with seizure disorders. The question does not indicate the client is experiencing any type of seizure disorder or is withdrawing from the alcohol. Options #2 and #4 are not indicated in this situation.

MRSA:

Many cultures

Requires gowns, gloves and goggles

Social isolation

Active infection

GLOVES:

Gloves

Lather up

Orifices

Very special handling

Everyone may be infected

Sharps

3.20 ② Option # 2 is the correct answer. Appropriate body mechanics is not bending at the waist. This may result in injury to the UAP. Options #1, #3, and #4 are incorrect for this clinical situation.

3.21 ④ Option #4 is the correct answer. Application of restraints is the last

intervention. Option #1 would be appropriate care for this client. Options #2 and #3 would also be appropriate care for this client.

COMBAT

Control immediate situation

Out of situation

Maintain calm

Be firm and set limits

Avoid restraints

Try consequences

3.22 ④ Answer is #4 based on CDC standards for this contamination. Options #1, #2, and #3 are incorrect for this contamination.

3.23 ③ Option #3 is the correct answer. The number one complication with safety for older adults is from medications. Options #1, #2, and #4 are incorrect.

3.24 ④ Option #4 is the correct answer. This should **NEVER** be done due to safety issues. The other options are not always a priority based on the type of equipment. Option #4 is always correct.

3.25 ③ Option #3 is the correct answer. This is too much oxygen for a client with this condition. Options #1, #2, and #4 are not answering the question related to the actual order for this client.

3.26 ① Option #1 is the correct answer. There is a risk for hypersensitivity to Ancef if there was a previous allergic reaction to Penicillin. The other options do not answer the question as it is currently written. (*Pharmacology Made Insanely Easy*, Manning & Rayfield)

I CAN HINT: "CEF" the GIANT will help you remember the major undesirable effects from cephalosporins. Remember these drugs start with a "*cef or ceph*"

GI distress

Increase in glucose values

Anaphylaxis to penicillin, **a**lcohol may cause vomiting

Nephrotoxicity

Thrombocytopenia

3.27 ①⑤ Options #1 and #5 are the correct answers. Option #2 should be squeezed directly onto the sterile field. Option #3 has contaminated gloves as currently reads. Sterile gloves should be placed on after unsterile bottle has been manipulated. Option #4 should be sterile gauze pad. Avoid using cotton balls because they may shed fibers in the wound, causing irritation, infection, or adhesion. Option #6 should be cleansed last since most drainage promotes bacterial growth. This drain is considered to be the most contaminated area.

3.28 ①③ Options #1 and #3 are the correct answer. Airway is a priority after a seizure. Do not attempt to force anything into the client's mouth if jaws are clenched shut. If jaws are not clenched, place an airway in client's mouth. This protects the tongue and also provides a method of suctioning the airway should the client vomit. Evaluate respiratory status. If vomiting occurs, be prepared to suction the client to clear the airway and prevent aspiration. Options #2, #4, and #5 are not necessary to have at the bedside for this client.

3.29 ④ Option #4 is the correct answer. Clean gloves should be worn at all times when handling any client's blood or body fluids. Option #1 is correct, but not a higher priority over #4. Option #2 is incorrect because venipuncture sites of client with hepatitis B should be held for a longer period of time due to possibility of increased bleeding associated with an impaired liver. Option #3 is incorrect standard of practice for used needles.

3.30 ②⑥ Options #2 and #6 are correct for this infection control procedure. Options #1 and #3 are correct for airborne transmission-based precautions. Option #4 should read "discard needles intact immediately after use into an impervious disposal box." Option #5 is not necessary. This would be appropriate for contact transmission-based precautions.

3.31 ② Option #2 is the correct answer. Intact rubber caps should be present on walker legs to prevent accidents. Options #1, #3, and #4 should be avoided for 4-6 weeks.

3.32 ③ Option #3 is the correct answer. Other options are incorrect, and do not reflect the standard of practice for this procedure.

3.33 ④ Option #4 is the correct answer. It includes options #1, #2, and #3.

3.34 ② Option #2 is the correct answer. Toothbrushes should not be shared due to the mode of transmission of HIV. Option #1 should be kept up to date. Option #3 should be wiped up with paper towel; the area should then be washed with soap and water and rinsed with Bleach and water and allowed to air. Option #4 is not correct since hands should be washed with soap and water.

3.35 ③ Option #3 is the correct answer since the client with insufficient parathyroid hormone may lead to a low calcium level. This can result in tetany, leading to possible seizures. Option #1 would be appropriate for a client with low thyroid, but is inappropriate for this condition. Option #2 would be appropriate for hyperthyroidism. Option #4 is not appropriate for this condition.

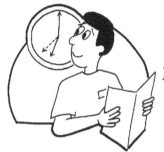 *Hey! Why don't you take a break!*

CHAPTER 4

Health Promotion and Maintenance

To keep the body in good health is a duty ... otherwise
we shall not be able to keep our mind strong and clear.
—Buddha

✔ Clarification of this test ...

The minimum standard includes performing and directing activities that promote and maintain the health of client/family. This includes growth and development through the aging process, disease prevention, health promotion programs, ante/intra/postpartum/ newborn care and immunizations. Activities in this chapter are not as heavily weighted as many of the activities in pharmacology or management. Activities that may be tested in this chapter include:

- ☛ Provide care that meets the needs of the newborn less than 1 month old through the infant or toddler client through 2 years
- ☛ Provide care that meets the needs of the preschool, school-age, and adolescent client ages 3 through 17 years
- ☛ Provide care that meets the needs of the adult client ages 18 through 64 years
- ☛ Provide care that meets the needs of the adult client ages 65 through 85 years and over
- ☛ Assist with fetal-heart monitoring for the antepartum client
- ☛ Assist with monitoring a client in labor
- ☛ Monitor recovery of stable postpartum client
- ☛ Assist with monitoring a client in labor
- ☛ Monitor recovery of stable postpartum client
- ☛ Collect data for health history
- ☛ Collect baseline physical data (i.e., skin integrity, and height and weight)
- ☛ Recognize barriers to communication and learning
- ☛ Compare client development to norms
- ☛ Assist client with expected life transition (i.e., attachment to newborn, parenting or retirement)
- ☛ Provide care and resources for beginning-of-life and/or end-of-life issues and choices
- ☛ Identify clients in need of immunizations (required and voluntary)
- ☛ Participate in health screening or health promotion programs
- ☛ Provide information for prevention of high-risk behaviors or lifestyle choices

---

4.1 Which of these recommendations should be included in a health-promotion session for women experiencing stress incontinence? *Select all that apply.*

① Reduce fluid intake to 400–600 mL/day.
② Carry and wear incontinence pads when at home and away from home
③ Discuss that incontinence is always secondary to an infection.
④ Review how to perform Kegel exercises.
⑤ Reduce the intake of tea, coke, and alcoholic beverages.

4.2 A geriatric client, newly diagnosed with diabetes, is being discharged. Client is alert, oriented, and able to independently maintain activities of daily living. Treatment will consist of a 1,500-caloric diabetic diet, insulin, and regular exercise by walking 30 minutes a day. What is a priority concern at the time the client is discharged?

① Does the client have adequate vision and manual dexterity to administer own insulin?
② Does the client understand the impact diabetes will have on lifestyle?
③ Since the client is living alone, is there a need for Home Health Care to check on client daily?
④ Does the client understand how to perform daily urinary sugar and acetone determinations?

4.3 Which communication technique is appropriate for a nurse to implement when caring for a client with a hearing loss?

① Irrigate the ear with warm water to remove any wax obstruction.
② Always touch the client prior to speaking to him.
③ Encourage the client to purchase a hearing aid.
④ Stand in front of him and speak clearly and slowly.

4.4 In preparation for discharge of a client with arterial insufficiency and Raynaud's phenomenon, what is the priority to include when reinforcing the teaching plan that the RN initiated?

① Walk several times each day as part of an exercise routine.
② Keep the heat up, so that the environment is warm.
③ Wear thromboembolic disease (TED) hose during the day.
④ Use hydrotherapy for increasing oxygenation.

4.5 What statement made by the nurse to the frustrated mother of a 15-year-old hospitalized daughter indicates the nurse understands the reason the daughter does not want her mom helping with care and wants to be left alone?

① "The adolescent is attempting to establish an identity away from the parents, which is painful for the parent, and child, but is a normal part of growth and development."
② "The adolescent is not feeling well, and is probably just taking out frustration on the mother because it is safe."
③ "It is essential to support the autonomy of the client, and the mother should respect the client's wishes."
④ "The relationship between the parent and child is not relevant at this time, and the client's wishes of parental involvement must be assessed."

4.6 A mother of a 2-week-old infant calls the LPN at the pediatrician's office. The mother states, "My baby sleeps all the time. I thought babies were supposed to keep parents awake. Do you think something is wrong?" How should the LPN respond to the mother's concerns?

① "I will schedule you an appointment for next week."
② "It is normal for infants to sleep a great deal."
③ "Is your baby sleeping about 15 hours a day?"
④ "How many feedings does your baby receive a day?"

4.7 A client is being prepared to be discharged following a laparoscopic cholecystectomy. What information would be most important for the LPN to reinforce during the teaching plan that the RN had initiated, in order to minimize complications with bloating and abdominal discomfort?

① "It will be important for you to decrease your intake of vegetables."
② "It will be important for you to walk around your home and not just sit in a chair."
③ "Feel free to take the analgesic as needed to decrease discomfort."
④ "You may want to decrease any physical activity until the discomfort subsides."

4.8 As the LPN is making midnight rounds, an 86-year-old client complains that his feet are cold. Which nursing action should the nurse do first?

① Elevate the foot of the bed and rub the feet to increase circulation.
② Assess the feet for pulses and adequacy of circulation.
③ Fill up a hot water bottle, wrap it in a case, and place on the feet.
④ Provide a warm drink for client to assist with warmth and relaxation.

4.9 The LPN is caring for a 2-year-old who has been recently admitted to the hospital. While conducting an assessment of the child, the nurse asks the parents to describe how the child goes to bed at night. The parents state, "What does that have to do with anything?" What information should the LPN provide to the family?

① Rituals of the child will be incorporated into the routine of the child (as appropriate) to promote stability and consistency.
② Children in this age group are at a high risk for injury.
③ It is hard for toddlers to sleep in the hospital.
④ Parents' wishes need to be maintained while the child is in the hospital.

4.10 While interviewing a woman beginning to go through menopause, the nurse is most concerned when the client states:

① "I seem to be having heavier periods than before."
② "I need to follow a heart healthy diet."
③ "I am more emotional than ever."
④ "I am glad I don't need birth control."

4.11 Which assessment should be reported to the provider of care for a newborn?

① Acrocyanosis and edema of the scalp.
② Head circumference of 40 cm.
③ Chest circumference of 32 cm.
④ Heart rate of 160 and respirations of 40.

4.12 What would be the priority of care for a client with Stage 2 Alzheimer's Disease who becomes agitated and refuses to answer further questions during an interview?

① Ask client if questions are upsetting in any way.
② Discontinue the interview.
③ Explain that the questions are necessary to complete plan of care.
④ Give client a small break and reconvene in five minutes.

4.13 Which statement by the parents indicates a need for further teaching about newborn care? "We will notify the provider of care for:

① more than one episode of projectile vomiting."
② absence of breathing for 10 seconds."
③ a temperature greater than 101 degrees F."
④ several liquid stools in 1 hour."

4.14 Which of the neonates in the newborn nursery should be assessed first?

① A 48-hour-neonate with a heart rate of 180 BPM when sleeping.
② A 14-hour neonate with RR- 45 breaths per minute and irregular.
③ A 24-hour neonate who has a bulging fontanel when crying.
④ A 2-week-old neonate who has seedy yellow stools after breastfeeding.

4.15 The LPN is obtaining vital signs on a young woman who is 26 weeks pregnant. Which statement made by the client would be of the greatest concern to the LPN?

① "I have more energy now than I did a few months ago."

② "My feet get a little swollen when I stand up at work for a long time."

③ "I think my body looks disgusting."

④ "My prenatal vitamin sometimes makes me nauseous."

4.16 The new parents of a young child are distraught when told by the physician that the child has an illness that will require the child be hospitalized for antibiotic therapy. Once admitted to the hospital, it is essential that the nurse:

① Encourages and demonstrates to the parents how to be involved in the child's care.

② Performs as much care for the child as possible to reduce the parent's stress.

③ Reviews the treatment course with the parents.

④ Determines the reason the child became ill in the first place.

4.17 The nurse is teaching a health promotion class to a group of high school girls. The nurse is providing instruction to the student on breast self-examination. Which statement made by the nurse is incorrect?

① "Perform the exam on the first day of your period, so you will remember."

② "Palpate the breast in any pattern you are comfortable with, remembering to cover the entire breast."

③ "It is important to perform the examination monthly to determine if any changes have occurred."

④ "You can examine your breasts in the shower."

4.18 The nurse is performing health screening examinations at the local high school. Which finding made by the LPN would be of greatest concern when examining a young man? The client:

① uses condoms.

② has tried smoking, but did not like it.

③ plays outdoor sports, but has never used sunscreen.

④ has a few friends.

4.19 The nurse is interviewing a young college student. The student admits to the nurse, "I had sex once or twice without a condom, but, the person I had sex with was not sick." How should the nurse respond to the client's statement?

① Inform client that most people with a sexually transmitted disease (STD) do not appear ill.

② Recommend the client be tested for HIV.

③ Teach the client about STD transmission and the importance of prevention.

④ Obtain the names of the individuals to call them and recommend STD screening.

4.20 A mother has brought a school aged child to the clinic for immunizations. Which statement made by the mother would require further assessment prior to the administration of the vaccinations?

① "My child is behind on vaccinations, but we will catch up."

② "My child had a cold three weeks ago."

③ "My child is afraid of the shots."

④ "My child cannot eat eggs."

4.21 A very anxious young mother says to the nurse, "I don't understand why you give my baby so many shots. Can't you just mix the medicine in one syringe and give one shot?" How can the nurse reassure the mother?

① "Unfortunately the vaccinations cannot be mixed. I will administer the medications as quickly as possible, and give you some ice to put on the site afterward."

② "Unfortunately, the vaccinations cannot be mixed. Children forget the pain of shots easily, so it will be okay."

③ "No, vaccinations cannot be mixed together. You will need to assist holding your child while they receive the injections."

④ "No, vaccinations cannot be mixed together. Would you like to leave the room while your child is vaccinated?"

4.22 The nurse is speaking to a junior high school health class about disease prevention. What information would be most important to include in the teaching plan:

① the effects of current lifestyle choices on later health
② that junior high school kids are healthy, and need to be kids
③ the importance of avoiding chocolate to prevent acne
④ the benefits of becoming a nurse to help educate the community

4.23 Which of these questions is the highest priority for the nurse when discussing safety for a 4-year-old with the parents?

① "Do you have all of your kitchen cabinets locked?"
② "Do the parents in your neighborhood feel comfortable reporting strangers?"
③ "Are you able to discuss your child's disagreements while playing with his friends to other parents?"
④ "Does your child have appropriate safety equipment for the games he plays?"

4.24 What question would be most important to ask a male client who is in for a digital rectal examination?

① "Have you noticed a change in the force of the urinary stream?"
② "Have you noticed a change in tolerance of certain foods in your diet?"
③ "Do you notice polyuria in the A.M.?"
④ "Do you notice any burning with urination or any odor to the urine?"

4.25 Which of these clients should the nurse question administering the influenza immunization?

① A 60-year-old who lives in an assisted living apartment.
② A 50-year-old who has a history of angina.
③ A 40-year-old who is allergic to iodine.
④ A 30-year-old who is allergic to eggs.

4.26 A client at 38 weeks gestation is admitted in active labor. The nursing assessment reveals a decreased blood pressure to 90/50 and FHR is 130 and regular. Which nursing action would be most important?

① Call the physician and advise of the decrease in blood pressure.
② Elevate the head of the bed to facilitate respirations.
③ Check the client's blood pressure and FHT every 30 minutes for the next 2 hours.
④ Place the client on left side and reevaluate the blood pressure.

4.27 During a 6-month-old well-baby check-up, what would the nurse expect on assessment?

① Pincer grasp
② Sit with support
③ Birth weight tripled
④ Presence of the posterior fontanelle

4.28 An elderly client with mild osteoarthritis needs instruction on exercising. In planning nursing care, which instruction would best help this client?

① Swimming is the only helpful exercise for osteoarthritis.
② Warm-up exercises should be done prior to exercising.
③ Exercises should be done routinely even if joint pain occurs.
④ Isometric exercises are most helpful to prevent contractures.

4.29 A physician orders an analgesic to be administered to a woman in labor who is 9 cm dilated and having contractions every 3 minutes lasting for 50 seconds. Which nursing action would be most important?

① Identify client prior to administering medication.
② Calculate the amount of medicine to be administered.
③ Hold the medication and document in nursing notes.
④ Notify the physician regarding the status of the contractions.

4.30 The nurse is caring for a client in labor. The nurse palpates a firm round form in the uterine fundus. On the client's right side, small parts are palpated, and on the left side, a long, smooth curved section is palpated. Which location should the nurse auscultate the fetal heart?

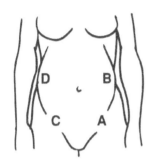

4.31 Which statement indicates a client understands how to safely breast-feed her newborn?

① "My baby will rest at least 7 hours between feedings."
② "My baby will feed approximately 9 minutes per feeding."
③ "My baby should have at least one bowel movement per day."
④ "My baby should have at least 7 to 8 wet diapers per day."

4.32 While preparing care for an elderly client with dementia, which plan is a priority?

① Encourage dependency with activities of daily living.
② Provide flexibility in schedules due to mental confusion.
③ Speak slowly and in a face-to-face position.
④ Limit reminiscing due to poor memory.

4.33 Which observation would most likely represent care-giver burnout in the daughter of an 80-year-old client with Alzheimer's?

① Failure of daughter to get parent into wheelchair daily.
② Daughter remains involved in family's activities.
③ Husband is seen assisting in mother-in-law's care.
④ Home environment extremely cluttered at each visit.

4.34 During the comprehensive history, the client reports an allergy to bananas, kiwis, and avocados. What is the most important question to ask during this assessment stage?

① "Do you have any problems with muscle cramps?"
② "Have you ever had any complications with latex allergy in the past?"
③ "Have you ever had any problems with diverticulosis?"
④ "Do you take a multiple vitamin?"

4.35 During the newborn assessment, the nurse is evaluating the rooting reflex. Locate where the nurse would stroke to elicit this response.

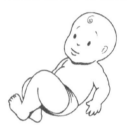

ANSWERS & RATIONALES

4.1 ④ Options #4 and #5 are correct. Option #4
⑤ will assist in strengthening the sphincter and structural supports of the bladder. Option #5 should be included because dietary irritants and natural diuretics, such as caffeine and alcoholic beverages, may increase stress incontinence. Option #1 is incorrect. If clients are non-restricted to the fluid intake, they should have a fluid intake of at least 2 to 3 L/day. Clients with stress incontinence may reduce their fluid intake to avoid incontinence at the risk of developing dehydration and urinary tract infection. This needs to be discouraged! Option #2 is incorrect. It would be more effective for a client to establish a voiding schedule that is regular than to carry incontinent pads. Option #3 is an incorrect statement. While a NEW symptom of incontinence may definitely occur in older clients if they have a UTI, the option reads "always" which does not take into account the numerous reasons for incontinence which are addressed in the hint below.

 I CAN HINT: The key to success in answering this question is to understand the cause of stress incontinence. We will review three types of urinary incontinence to assist you with this process.

Stress Incontinence: Relaxed pelvic floor musculature, atrophy due to loss of estrogen resulting in small amount of urine loss during coughing, sneezing, laughing, or other physical activities, continuous leak at rest or with minimal exertion (e.g., postural changes).

Urge: Involuntary detrusor (bladder) contractions (DI), along with sphincter relaxation. Seen with CNS disorders (Parkinson's disease); bladder disorders (interstitial cystitis). Signs and symptoms include loss of urine with an abrupt and strong desire to void; involuntary loss of urine (without symptoms); nocturia is common.

Functional: Chronic functional and mental disabilities. Urge incontinence or functional limitations or environmental factors.

4.2 ① Option #1 is correct. It is very important that the geriatric client have the visual and manual skills to administer the insulin. Options #2 and #3 are important to determine; but option #1 is a priority. Option #4, urinary tests are not commonly used to monitor diabetes.

 I CAN HINT: "MAKE" will assist you in evaluating if an elderly client is competent to administer insulin to self.

Manual dexterity

Adequate vision

Kogntive (Cognitive) ability

Evaluate signs and symptoms of hyper and hypoglycemia

4.3 ④ Option #4 is correct. The nurse should always stand in front of the hearing-impaired client, and raising the voice is not as effective as clear, slow speech. Option #1 is not necessary since there is no indication of cerumen being impacted. Option #2 is incorrect because it is important that a sensory-impaired client be aware of someone's presence before they are touched. The best way to get their attention is by raising your hand or arm. Option #3 may be appropriate at a later time; however, his care needs to be addressed at the present.

 I CAN HINT: Hearing loss is very common in older adult clients. Questions about hearing loss may be incorporated with other questions related to chronic health problems. "HEARING" will assist you in organizing nursing interventions for a client with hearing impairment.

Hearing aid is taught how to care for it

Evaluate how to remove ear wax if impacted cerumen is a problem; may need an ear irrigation

Assess for dizziness, nausea, and vomiting if had a stapedectomy

Reassure client during communication by standing in front of client at eye level to speak; speak slowly

Instruct client not to wear hearing aid while bathing or swimming

No hair spray, cosmetics, or oils around ear

Give hearing aid a rest at night and turn it off and open the battery compartment to prevent battery drain

4.4 ② Option#2 is correct. Raynaud's phenomenon consists of intermittent episodic spasms of the arterioles, most frequently in the fingers and toes. Symptoms are precipitated by exposure to cold, emotional upset, or nicotine and caffeine intake. The client's instructions should include keeping the environment warm to prevent vasoconstriction. Wearing gloves, warm clothes, and socks will also be useful in preventing vasoconstriction, (option #3) but TED hose would not be therapeutic. Option #1 is incorrect. Walking will most likely increase pain. Option #4 is incorrect. Spasms are not necessarily correlated with other peripheral vascular problems.

 I CAN HINT: "STRESS" will assist you in remembering what to reinforce in the teaching that was initiated for the client in order to prevent vasospasm.

Stress management

The hands, feet, nose, and ears need to be protected when exposed to cold weather

Refrigerated or freezer objects—client should wear gloves when handling

Environment needs to be warm

Stress the importance of avoiding caffeine

Stress the importance of avoiding tobacco products

4.5 ① Option #1 is correct. This question is evaluating your understanding of how to "provide education that meets the special needs of specific ages." The adolescent is struggling to accomplish the developmental task of "Identity versus Role Diffusion." The 15-year-old wants to be independent, and with the trauma of being hospitalized the adolescent may be even working harder to do things independently. The mother needs to understand this is part of this stage of development. With appropriate knowledge, the mother will have the tools to also support her daughter during this stage of development even after the daughter is discharged from the hospital. Option #2 is incorrect. Even though there may be some validity to this statement, it is not the actual rationale for the psychological development for the daughter. If the daughter's developmental needs are being addressed, there will be no need to get frustrated. Option #3 does not address the mother's feelings of frustration. This option only makes a statement and does not provide any rationale as to the reason for the behavior. Option #4 totally ignores the needs of the mother. In every relationship there are 2 people involved. In order to meet the daughter's needs, the mother needs to understand the behavior.

 I CAN HINT: "PAIRS" will assist you in organizing concepts for the adolescent when answering questions in the future.

Peer group

Altered body image

Identity - Independent

Role diffusion

Separation from peers

4.6 ④ Option #4 is correct as it is essential to determine if the newborn is receiving enough calories and fluid intake to promote growth. The nurse needs to evaluate if the mother is waking the newborn for feedings. Option #1 is not appropriate, as the LPN has not made an assessment of the situation to determine if / when an appointment is necessary, not enough information to obtain a recommendation from the physician. Option #2 does not address the mother's concern, nor assesses the situation. Option #3 is incorrect as newborns sleep approximately 20 hours a day.

4.7 ② Option #2 is the correct answer. This discomfort may be caused by "free air" which is a result of CO_2. This will be absorbed by ambulation. It is important for the client to walk and not remain in the chair. Option #1 is incorrect. There is no indication for this. Option #3 is not a priority. In reality, there is less need for pain medication with the laparoscopic procedure. Option #4 is incorrect.

4.8 ② Option #2 is the correct answer. Assessment must be done prior to implementation. The client may have decreased circulation that has increased in severity over the past few hours. Options #1 and #3 would be contraindicated. Option #4 would be secondary.

4.9 ① Option #1 is the correct answer. Toddlers thrive on rituals and routines and by incorporating these into the care of the child, the impact of the hospitalization will hopefully be minimized. Option #2 is true, but the nurse is inquiring about routines, not injury prevention. Option #3 does not provide the needed information to the parents. Most people of any age have difficulty sleeping in the hospital. Option #4 is incorrect, as the nurse is supporting the growth and development of the child, not the parents' wishes.

I CAN HINT: "PRAISE" will assist you in organizing concepts for toddler care.

Push-pull toys, Parallel play

Rituals and Routines, Regression,

Autonomy versus shame and doubt, Accidents

Involve parents

Separation anxiety

Elimination, Explore

4.10 ④ Option #4 is the correct answer. Options #1, #2, and #3 are normal findings of a menopausal woman. The concerning statement is option #4. Although the woman is beginning to go through menopause, this does not mean fertility is lost. Menopause may take several years to complete, so it is essential that the woman understands that an absence or irregular period does not guarantee birth control is not necessary.

4.11 ② Option #2 is the correct answer. Average circumference of the head for a neonate ranges between 32 to 36 cm. An increase in size may indicate hydrocephaly or increased intracranial pressure. Options #1, #3, and #4 are normal newborn assessments.

4.12 ② The correct answer is option #2. It would be the most appropriate response due to the agitation and refusal to answer questions. The client may be getting overwhelmed. Option #1 is incorrect. The behavior of the client demonstrates that these questions are upsetting the client. Option #3 does not answer the question. The question indicates the client is becoming agitated and refuses to answer further questions. The answer needs to address the problem the client is experiencing verses what the nurse needs to get accomplished. Option #4 is not correct since this time frame will not allow the client to regroup.

4.13 ② Option #2 is the correct answer. This is a normal newborn assessment and should not be reported. Option #1 should be reported, so there is no need for further teaching. The newborn may spit up, but if there are multiple episodes of projectile vomiting, then there may be a physiological problem such as pyloric stenosis. Option #3 should also be reported since this temperature may indicate a complication with sepsis. Option #4 may indicate a complication and could result in alteration in fluid and electrolytes.

4.14 ① Option #1 is the correct answer. The neonate's HR should be between 120 – 160 BPM. When the neonate is crying the HR will increase, but when asleep the HR of 180 BPM is way too high. Option #2 is not a complication. RR of a neonate typically is between 30–50. Option #3 is an expected finding when a neonate is crying. Option #4 is an expected finding when a neonate is breastfeeding.

4.15 ③ Option #3 is the correct answer. Option #3 is the greatest concern as this statement indicates the client is not psychologically adjusting to the physical changes of pregnancy, and further evaluation of these feelings is necessary. Option #1 is a common finding. Women in the second trimester of pregnancy often feel an increase in their energy level. Option #2 is not uncommon. Many women (pregnant or not) will have slight swelling in their feet when standing / sitting for long periods. Option #4 is common. Prenatal vitamins often can upset a woman's stomach, and need to be instructed on methods to decrease this side effect.

4.16 ① Option #1 is the correct answer. It is important to support the parents and encourage them to remain involved with the day to day activities of the child. Parents are often fearful, feel a lack of control, and are anxious when a child is ill. Option #2 is incorrect. The nurse should perform tasks the parents are unwilling or unable to perform, but should allow and encourage the parents to be involved as possible. Option #3 is the role of the physician. Option #4 is inappropriate for the situation presented in the question.

4.17 ① Option #1 is the correct answer. Women often have breast tenderness associated with menstruation, so it is recommended that women do not perform BSE while menstruating. Options #2, #3, and #4 are correct statements, but the question is asking for the incorrect statement.

4.18 ③ Option #3 is the correct answer. The lack of sunscreen use puts the client at high risk to develop skin cancer in the future. By intervening now, and encouraging the use of sunscreen, the LPN can help prevent concerns in the future. Option #1 may be of concern, but the young man is practicing safer sex by using condoms. Option #2 is not of concern, as the client did not continue smoking. Option #4 is incorrect, as it is important for teenagers to have friends.

4.19 ③ Option #3 is the correct answer. This provides the client with information which could help reduce the risks associated with unprotected sex. Option #1 provides information, but does not teach the client. Option #2 would be appropriate, but without teaching the client about disease transmission, it is unlikely the client will change the high risk behavior, or seek testing. Option #4 is not within the scope of the nurse. This is the job of the health department once an individual has been diagnosed.

4.20 ④ Option #4 is the correct answer. This is concerning as an allergy to eggs or gelatin should be reported to the physician, so the physician can determine if the vaccination should be given. Option #1 is a positive statement made by the mother. The mother is recognizing the fact the vaccines are behind, and is planning to catch up. Option #2 is not clinically significant, as the child is not currently ill. Option #3 is normal for children.

4.21 ① Option #1 is the correct answer. It is not uncommon for parents, and children, to be anxious regarding injections. By informing the mother that vaccines cannot be mixed, assuring her the shots will be given quickly, and offering an intervention the mother can comfort the child afterward. This would be the best way to decrease the mother's anxiety. Option #2 is untrue, children do not forget shots. Options #3 and #4 do not reassure the mother.

4.22 ① Option #1 is the correct answer. The lifestyle choices of this age group, (diet/smoking/exercise) or lack thereof, will impact the individuals later health. For example, a 14-year-old that smokes is unlikely to experience symptoms until later on in life, such as 25 years of age. An overweight teen is unlikely to have co-mortifies, such as HTN; however, later in life these co-morbities can be expected. Options #2, #3, and #4 are incorrect as they do not deal with disease prevention.

4.23 ④ Option #4 is the correct answer. It is the priority due to the developmental stage of the 4-year-old child. The 4-year-old is very active and safety is most important. Option #1 would be a priority for the toddler. Options #2 and #3 are important, but not a priority.

4.24 ① Option #1 is correct. This change would be most indicative of a potential complication with (BPH) benign prostate hypertrophy. Options #2, #3, and #4 are incorrect. Option #4 would be indicative of an infection.

4.25 ④ Option #4 is the correct answer. If a client is allergic to eggs, there is a risk for allergies to the influenza immunization as well. Option # 1 does not address the question. Option #2 is not correct for this question. Option #3 would be appropriate for clients who were going to experience a diagnostic procedure that used dyes.

4.26 ④ Option #4 is the correct answer. The decrease in blood pressure is most likely due to pressure on the inferior vena cava which occurs in the supine position (vena-caval syndrome). By positioning the client on left side, the pressure is relieved and blood pressure should increase. Option #1 may be necessary, but option #4 should be done first. Option #2 does not address the problem of low blood pressure. Option #3 is not correct because the current problem needs to be addressed immediately.

4.27 ② Option #2 is the correct answer. A 6-month-old should sit with help. Option #1 is present at 9 months of age. Option #3 is present at 1 year. Option #4 is not correct because it should be closed by 2-3 months.

4.28 ② Option #2 is correct. Warm-up or stretching exercises should always be done prior to and after exercising. Option #1 is only one helpful exercise. Option #3 is incorrect because painful joints should not be exercised. Option #4 does not involve joint movements.

4.29 ④ Option #4 is the correct answer. The information indicates the woman is in the transition phase. Analgesics could cause depressed respirations in the baby. Options #1 and #2 contain correct information, but not for this situation. Option #3 does not address the immediate problem.

4.30 The fetal heart rate with the LOA position would be auscultated at point A. LOP–point B; ROA–point C; ROP–point D.

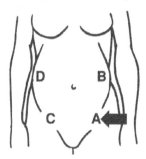

4.31 ④ Option #4 is the correct answer. This indicates the baby is ingesting an appropriate amount of nutrition. Option #1 is incorrect. Newborns feed approximately every 2-3 hours during the day and every 4 hours during the night. Option #2 is incorrect. The newborn should nurse for approximately 15-20 minutes per breast. Option #3 is incorrect. The newborn should have at least 2 bowel movements daily.

4.32 ③ Option #3 is correct. This is most effective when communicating with an elderly client. Option # 1 is incorrect because independence is encouraged. Option #2 is incorrect because schedules need to be routine, reinforce, and repeated. Flexibility leads to confusion. Option #4 is incorrect because reminiscing helps the client resume progression through the grief process associated with disappointing life events and increases self-esteem.

4.33 ④ Option #4 is the correct answer. Option #4 is correct as this may represent depression and burnout. Option #1 may be impossible for daughter to do alone. Options #2 and #3 are very healthy and desirable.

4.34 ② Option #2 is the correct answer. Clients who have allergies to these foods (bananas, kiwis and avocados) typically are high risk for latex allergy due to the cross reactivity of the proteins present in these fruits and latex. Options #1, #3, and #4 are incorrect.

4.35

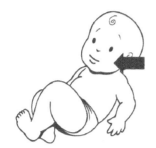

CHAPTER 5
Psychosocial Integrity

The brain is wider than the sky.
—Emily Dickenson

✔ Clarification of this test ...

The minimum standard includes performing and directing activities related to caring for client / family with emotional, mental and social problems including behavioral interventions.

- ☛ Assist in or reinforce education to caregivers/family on ways to manage client with behavioral disorders
- ☛ Participate in behavior management program by recognizing environmental stressors and/or providing a therapeutic environment
- ☛ Participate in reminiscence therapy, validation therapy or reality orientation
- ☛ Participate in client group session
- ☛ Identify signs and symptoms of substance abuse/chemical dependency, withdrawal or toxicity
- ☛ Collect data regarding client's psychosocial functioning
- ☛ Identify client use of effective and ineffective coping mechanisms
- ☛ Identify stressors that may affect recovery/health maintenance (i.e., lifestyle, body changes, environmental)
- ☛ Assist client to cope/adapt to stressful events and changes in health status (i.e., abuse/neglect, end of life, grief and loss, life changes or physical changes)
- ☛ Collect data on client's potential for violence to self and others
- ☛ Assist in managing the care of angry/agitated client (i.e., de-escalation techniques)
- ☛ Make adjustment to care with consideration of client's spiritual and cultural beliefs
- ☛ Explore why client is refusing or not following treatment plan
- ☛ Assist in the care of a client experiencing sensory/perceptual alterations
- ☛ Assist in the care of the cognitively impaired client
- ☛ Promote positive self-esteem of client
- ☛ Promote emotional support to client and family
- ☛ Use therapeutic communication techniques with client

5.1 What is the priority nursing action for a client who throws the lunch tray and yells that nobody cares for her and starts to become combative?

① Remove the client from the lunch room.
② Try to gain client's trust.
③ Speak strongly and ask client to stop.
④ Administer client the PRN medication.

5.2 What would be the priority of care for a client who is experiencing a manic episode and starting to become combative?

① Assist the client to the recreation room for a game of pool.
② Escort client to a quiet room with no other people or activities occurring.
③ Encourage client to verbalize thoughts and feelings.
④ Set firm limits on client's behavior and expectations.

5.3 Which one of these statements made by an adolescent client with anorexia nervosa is a priority for immediate intervention by the nurse?

① "I know that the reason I do not have any friends is because I am ugly and fat."
② "Today I am feeling faint and weak."
③ "I am experiencing some tenderness with my mouth when I brush my teeth."
④ "I am not thin enough."

5.4 What should be the priority plan of care for the LPN who says "I do not want to be the nurse for this client" after receiving the assignment for a client with Kaposi's sarcoma and pneumocystis carinii?

① Change the LPN's assignment.
② Provide a reference regarding Standard Precautions.
③ Provide assistance with the assignment.
④ Respond by saying, "You act worried about this assignment."

5.5 During the planning sessions for a group of clients who have been diagnosed with chronic diseases, the nurse demonstrates an understanding of the reason religious involvement may contribute to successful coping by the client when the nurse states the following? *Select all that apply.* "Religious involvement has been known to:

① reduce psychological stress."
② buffer against depression."
③ speed recovery from emotional disorders."
④ reduce the immune system."
⑤ increase phagocytosis."

5.6 The LPN makes a home visit to an elderly client that lives alone. The client states to the LPN, "My children have planned for me to move to an assisted living facility. I don't want to go. They didn't even ask me if I wanted to move." How should the LPN respond?

① "I am sure your children have your best interest in mind."
② "It seems like you are sad."
③ "Why don't you want to move?"
④ "What was your children's response when you told them how you felt?"

5.7 The nurse is working for a hospice agency, and is assigned the care of an 11 year-old-client. The client says to the nurse, "My parents are sad and think this is their fault, but, I know it is my fault." How should the nurse proceed?

① Discuss the conversation with the parents.
② Notify the field supervisor of the situation.
③ Ask the child what makes him feel that way.
④ Recognize this is normal growth and development.

5.8 A client of Native American heritage is admitted to the hospital with a diagnosis of Crohn's disease. Although the client is compliant with the medical treatment, the client informs the nurse that, "My tribe's medicine man is coming in to assist in my healing." The medicine man arrives with a tonic and herbal solution for the client to drink. How should the LPN proceed?

  ① Allow the client to consume the tonic.
  ② Ask the medicine man what is in the tonic and consult with the physician and pharmacy of possible interactions.
  ③ Educate the client and medicine man about the benefits of Western medicine.
  ④ Ask the charge nurse to assist with removing the medicine man from the room.

5.9 A client is in the doctor's office after receiving a diagnosis of cancer with a poor prognosis. The client expresses concern that tubes and wires will be placed to keep him alive. What could the nurse recommend to assist the client?

  ① Discuss fears and concerns with the family and fill out an advanced directive.
  ② Discuss fears and concerns with the physician.
  ③ Consult an attorney to draw a will.
  ④ Discuss feelings with their pastor.

5.10 The nurse is performing an assessment on an elderly client with dementia, who is accompanied by a caregiver. What statement made by the caregiver would be of greatest concern to the nurse?

  ① "I am arranging for assistance from the church."
  ② "I put chairs in front of the doors."
  ③ "I have respite care come twice a week."
  ④ "I need a break from all this."

5.11 A nurse is visiting the home of a young woman, who has suffered from severe depression since the recent death of her husband. The house is matted, the kitchen is dirty, and the children are in pajamas watching TV. The nurse is concerned that:

  ① The client's depression may lead to a suicide attempt.
  ② The client's depression may be causing neglect to the children.
  ③ The client's depression would improve if the home were cleaned.
  ④ The client's depression would improve with anti-depressant therapy.

5.12 Which nursing action would be most appropriate in helping an elderly, depressed, client complete activities of daily living?

  ① Medicate client prior to any activity.
  ② Assist client with grooming in order to save time.
  ③ Provide frequent forceful direction to keep the client focused.
  ④ Develop a written schedule of activities, allowing extra time.

5.13 The nurse is working at a psychiatric facility. A client is constantly ambulating in the hallway, and stating, "I am the president, get out of my way." Based on this finding, what would an appropriate intervention be for this client?

  ① Take the client outside for a lengthy walk.
  ② Encourage the client to play cards.
  ③ Obtain a sandwich for the client.
  ④ Inform the client he is not the president, and take him to his room.

5.14 The nurse is approached by a friend and states, "I am so concerned about my son. He is so depressed. I don't know what to do. Can you help me?" The nurse is agreeable to assist the friend, and is aware of the importance to find out if:

  ① The son has made statements regarding suicide.
  ② The son has had a recent loss in his life.
  ③ The son has good friends.
  ④ The son is taking drugs.

5.15 A client is scheduled to begin chemotherapy after a recent mastectomy. The client states, "I already am disfigured; now I am going to be bald as well. This is not fair!" What response made by the nurse would be appropriate?

① "At least you will be alive, and your hair will grow back soon."

② "I know you will be able to get through this."

③ "I can't imagine how difficult this is for you. How are you handling everything?"

④ "My mother had cancer, and it was awful."

5.16 A new client comes to the physician's office for a routine physical. The nurse is interviewing the client, and the client states, "I am an alcoholic that has been in recovery for some time, and am new to the area. Do you have any information about the local AA?" What action should the nurse take?

① Provide the client with the phone numbers of facilities that have AA meetings.

② Inform the physician of the client's request.

③ Ask the client when he had his last drink.

④ Inform the client that he is at high risk to resume drinking.

5.17 The nurse is answering calls at the local crisis hotline. A young man calls in and says, "She left me, and this hurts so badly. I don't think I can live through this!" How should the nurse respond to the client?

① "How long have you felt this way?"

② "Do you have a plan to hurt yourself?"

③ "What happened that makes you feel this way?"

④ "What can be done to make you feel better?"

5.18 While eating dinner in the dining room, a client on a locked psychiatric unit suddenly throws their cup and screams, "I am getting out of here." What activities of the nurse are the most appropriate?

① Call security, and remove the other clients from the dining room.

② Remove objects within the client's reach, and calmly tell the client to leave the dining room immediately.

③ Have another nurse prepare a sedative, and remove the other clients from the dining area.

④ Give the client another cup, and tell them that behavior is inappropriate and unacceptable.

5.19 The LPN working for hospice receives a call that a client has expired. The nurse goes to the home of the client, and finds the client on the floor and surrounded by men of the family. How should the nurse proceed?

① Determine if it would be appropriate to assess the client at this time.

② Ask if the men could help the nurse get the client back into bed for an assessment.

③ Recognize this is abnormal, and notify the hospice supervisor.

④ Assess the environment to determine how the client fell to the floor.

5.20 The LPN is working for a hospice agency and is making a home visit to a client. The client says to the nurse, "I am ready for this, but my family is not. What can I do to help them?" The nurse's best response would be:

① "Your family loves you, and will never be ready."

② "Have you told them how you feel?"

③ "I will talk with them for you."

④ "Denial is a normal part of the grieving process."

5.21 The family member of a hospice client calls the nurse and state, "I think the end is close." Which assessment findings would indicate the statement is correct?

① decreased edema, 10 second periods of apnea, cool skin

② refusal of fluids, increased time sleeping, worsening of incontinence

③ Cheyne-Stokes respirations, diarrhea, increase in edema

④ increase in alertness, shallow respirations, anorexia

5.22 A client who has suffered an amputation after a car accident says to the nurse, "I know the surgery saved my life, and everyone says I am lucky, but I don't feel that way." What response should the nurse make?

① "You are lucky, and will get better with therapy."
② "I know this must be hard, but your family loves you, and will help you through this."
③ "You have suffered a loss, and it is okay to grieve."
④ "I am sure this has been difficult, do you want to see a counselor?"

5.23 During an appointment, the physician determines that an elderly client has a visual impairment that is significant enough to revoke the client's driver's license. The client says to the nurse, "I just can't believe this is happening to me. What am I going to do now?" The nurse can best respond to the client by:

① Asking if there is anyone the client would like to call.
② Allowing the client to express feelings.
③ Offering to call a taxi for the client.
④ Offering information of public transportation.

5.24 The LPN is working on a very busy medical surgical unit. The nurse had three admissions, a discharge, and a transfer to the ICU. While working on the third admission a family member of an assigned client says, "This has been a very busy night for you. I had planned on going home, but, I think I should stay." How should the nurse respond?

① "It has been a terribly busy night. I think that would be a good idea."
② "I am very busy, but I can handle it."
③ "It's another day in paradise."
④ "What makes you feel like you need to stay?"

5.25 An American Indian client is scheduled for a joint replacement. Upon admission for surgery, the client says to the nurse, "I need to have the tissues that are removed, so they can be buried with me when I die. Without them, I will not be whole in my afterlife." What action should the nurse take?

① Inform the client this request violates protocol.
② Inform the client this request does not make sense.
③ Inform the surgeon of the client's request.
④ Inform the operating room staff to save the tissue removed.

5.26 A client is admitted to the hospital, and is requesting a visit from the pastor of the church. The nurse has been assigned this client, and is to administer a timed medication. When the nurse enters the room, the client and the pastor are praying. What would be appropriate for the nurse to do at this time?

① Leave the room without interruption of the client and pastor.
② Administer the medication as quickly and quietly as possible.
③ Explain the reason for the interruption of the prayer process.
④ Notify the pharmacy that the time of the medication needs to be rescheduled.

5.27 A wife of a client with dementia says to the nurse, "It is hard to see my husband get so frustrated and angry when he tries to remember things. I just don't understand this." What teaching should the nurse provide to the spouse?

① "It is common. The dementia will cause him to forget the frustration and anger."
② "It is common for clients with dementia to become frustrated. How are you handling this?"
③ "Clients with dementia often suffer from frustration and anger when trying to perform tasks. It is important for you to take care of yourself in order to take care of him."
④ "Clients with dementia are difficult to care for at home. When you feel overwhelmed, it may be necessary to place your husband in a facility."

5.28 A post partum mother comes to the OB office for a routine follow up visit. Upon entering the room, the nurse finds the newborn in the car seat crying, and the post partum mother sitting in the chair looking away from the infant. Which statement made by the nurse would be the most therapeutic at this time?

① "Can I get your baby for you?"
② "Sometimes it is hard to adjust to becoming a new mother. How are you doing?"
③ "I know this must be difficult on you. Where is the baby's father?"
④ "You don't seem like you are doing too well with becoming a mother."

5.29 Which of these symptoms may be assessed for a client experiencing alcohol withdrawal? *Select all that apply.*

① HR–56 beats per minute.
② BP–102/68.
③ Fine tremor of both hands.
④ Vomiting.
⑤ Inability to sleep.

5.30 A mother of a one-year-old comes to the office for a routine examination. The woman reports to the nurse, "I am so stressed out lately. I am having a hard time managing everything, and I don't know how to make it better." What response made be the LPN is most helpful in evaluating the situation of the mother?

① "Has something changed in your life?"
② "Have you been suffering from post partum depression?"
③ "Why do you feel this way?"
④ "How can I help you make this better?"

5.31 Which of these psychiatric clients should be evaluated first?

① Depressed client sitting on the floor rocking back and forth.
② Bipolar client pacing and clenching fist.
③ Psychotic client who is having a delusion that she is the Queen of England.
④ Schizophrenic client laughing and waving hands up in the air.

5.32 A client has just been diagnosed with a terminal illness. When the nurse enters the room, the client is crying and states, "I can't believe this is happening to me". Which response made by the LPN is the most appropriate?

① Evaluate if the client understands the diagnosis.
② Determine if the client would like to have a member of the church visit.
③ Notify the physician of the client's response.
④ Remain silent and let the client make the next statement.

5.33 A client rings the call bell and is requesting assistance to ambulate to the bathroom. The LPN delegates this to the UAP. The UAP states, "I am so glad that I am the only one that is qualified to take someone to the bathroom. I guess they don't teach that in nursing school." How should the LPN respond?

① "That was rude."
② "You sound like you are upset about something."
③ "Ambulating clients to the bathroom is within your scope of practice."
④ "We all have things about our job we do not like."

5.34 A client with a history of schizophrenia is admitted to a surgical unit following a cholecystecomy. The client is agitated and says to the nurse, "Someone is trying to kill me! Get me out of here!" Which intervention by the LPN would be appropriate?

① Administer a tranquilizer stat.
② Notify the charge nurse of the client's concerns.
③ Move the client to a room close to the nurses' station for close observation.
④ Check the bathroom for intruders.

5.35 The nurse understands that a therapeutic nurse–client relationship is characterized by:

① Establishing priorities and goals for the client.
② Collaborating to establish mutually agreed upon goals and priorities.
③ Utilizing the nursing process to establish client goals.
④ Directing interactions to assist the client to meet needs.

ANSWERS & RATIONALES

5.1 ① Option #1 is the answer. It is important to remove the combative client from a setting where she might harm herself and others. Option #2 is important, but if she is yelling, it would not be the top priority. Option #3 is setting limits and is an appropriate second action. Option #4 would be last if all else fails.

I CAN HINT: The key to answering this question is to understand how to provide care for a client who becomes combative. "COMBAT" will assist you with these strategies for clinical thinking.

Control immediate situation
Out of situation
Maintain calmness
Be firm/set limits
Avoid restraints if possible
Try consequences

5.2 ② Option #2 is correct. This will assist client with establishing some control over behavior with no outside stimuli and activities for distraction. Option #1 would only contribute to the manic episode and would not be therapeutic. The last thing the nurse would want the client to engage in would be a competitive activity. Option #3 is incorrect. During the manic episode, the client is out of control and needs time to regroup. Option #4 is incorrect for the manic client. This would be appropriate if client was demonstrating manipulative behavior.

I CAN HINT: "COMBAT" will assist you in organizing your care for a client who is becoming combative. An easy way to think about this is to think about "time out" with a toddler who is acting out. The goal is to calm the client.

Control the immediate situation
Out of situation (remove client by escorting to quiet room or a quiet location)
Maintain a calm behavior
Be firm/set limits before becoming manic and combative
Avoid restraints if possible
Try consequences

5.3 ② Option #2 is correct. This client may be experiencing some alerations in fluid and electrolytes leading to cardiovascular complications. Option #1 is part of the reason the client has developed this disorder from the low self-esteem. Option #3 would not be a priority. It would be a concern but would not require immediate intervention. Option #4 is incorrect. This is very similar to Option #1 which are both symptoms of a low self esteem. Neither of these, however, would require immediate intervention.

I CAN HINT: The key to answering this correctly is to focus on the anorexia nervosa and the "immediate intervention." This indicates there is a complication that is an immediate threat to the client's safety. After clustering options #1 and #4 together, that would leave options #2 and #3 for the selection. While we would be concerned with option #3, the question to ask is "Would mouth tenderness cause an immediate threat to the client?" versus "Would a feeling of faint and weakness cause an immediate threat to the client?"

5.4 ④ Option #4 is the correct answer. This allows the LPN to ventilate concerns with this assignment. Options #1, #2, and #3 do not address the LPN's concerns, and consequently will not provide additional assessments as to the fear the LPN has. It is important to understand how to provide support in order to assist the LPN in feeling comfortable in accepting this assignment in the future.

I CAN HINT: This question is evaluating your ability to respond to the LPN and provide support through therapeutic communication. Strategies for therapeutic communication is to promote "**TRUST**".

Try expression of thoughts and feelings
Reflect
Use silence
Set limits
Time with client

5.5 ① Options # 1, #2, #3 are correct. *American*
② *Journal of Psychiatry* 1992, 149:1693-
③ 1700, l *American Journal of Psychiatry* 1998, 155:536-542; *Journal of Nervous and Mental Disease* 2007, 195: 389-395. From 2000–2008 140 of 223 studies (63%) reported less depression or faster recovery from depression in the more religious. Options #4 and # 5 are incorrect; there is no research supporting these facts.

5.6 ④ Option #4 is the correct answer. This is an open-ended response and will help to get the client to think about the importance of discussing feelings with the correct family members? This provides information to the LPN about the family situation through performing an assessment. Option #1 disregards the feelings of the client. Option #2 is inappropriate as there is no indication the client is sad or grieving. Option #3 does not address the client's feelings of not wanting to move.

5.7 ③ Option #3 is the correct answer. The nurse needs to establish a relationship with the client, regardless of age. The client identifies that the parents are having concerns regarding guilt, as well as the client. The nurse needs to explore the situation, and asking an open ended question would be helpful. Option #1 may be indicated, but not until the nurse has assessed the situation and determined why the child felt that way. Option #2 is not indicated. There is no evidence of abuse. Option #4 is untrue, as this is not normal growth and development.

5.8 ② Option #2 is the correct answer. The client should be allowed to incorporate culture into medical care using the SPIRIT method. (Refer to book: Nursing Made Insanely Easy, Rayfield & Manning) It is important for the nurse to know what is in the tonic and evaluate for herbal interactions with the medications the client is receiving. Option #1 is unsafe. The nurse needs to know what the client will be taking. Option #3 dismisses the belief of the client in the medicine man. Option #4 is inappropriate.

5.9 ① Option #1 is the correct answer. The client should discuss their wishes with their family and prepare an advance directive to guide treatment should the client become unable to make decisions. Option #2 is feasible, however, should the client not have an advance directive, then the physician cannot execute the client's wishes without the family's consent. Option #3 does not address the medical concerns the client has. Option #4 will not help resolve the issue of life support.

5.10 ④ Option #4 is the correct answer. This statement clearly indicates the care giver feels tired / overwhelmed. Caring for a client with dementia is extremely challenging, especially as the disease progresses. It would be important for the nurse at this point, to determine if the caregiver felt able to continue to care for the client, had a support system, and was able to take care of themselves (eating, sleeping, and socializing). A caregiver who cannot care for themselves will not be able to care for another. This client could be at risk for neglect. Options #1 and #3 indicate the caregiver is receiving assistance. Option #2 is a method to contain the person with dementia in the home. If attempting to move the chairs, the caregiver would hear the chairs being moved. Also, by placing the chair in front of the door, the person with dementia may not recognize that the door is behind the chair.

CHAPTER 5: ANSWERS & RATIONALES

5.11 ② Option #2 is the correct answer. A client with severe depression may not be able to care for themselves, let alone children. The fact that the children are not dressed, watching television, and the home is matted indicates the young woman may not be able to meet the needs of her children. Option #1 is not correct. A severe depression does not mean a suicide attempt will be made. Option #3 is incorrect. The client's depression will not improve with a clean home. Option #4 is incorrect. Nurses do not prescribe medications. The nurse could and should refer this client to a mental healthcare provider.

5.12 ④ Option #4 is the correct answer. A written schedule with built in extra-time will allow the client to understand what is expected and will allow her to participate at a slower speed. Option #1 is incorrect. This may not be necessary. Option #2 is incorrect. This may increase the client's dependency and may interfere with self esteem. Option #3 is incorrect. The nurse should not be forceful, but should be consistent with a structured plan.

5.13 ③ Option #3 is the correct answer. The constant ambulation, and grandiose delusion of being president, indicate the client suffers from bipolar disorder, and is in the manic phase of the disease. The client experiencing mania often does not stop, even to eat. It would be hard (if not impossible) for this client to sit at the table for a meal. The provision of finger foods by the nurse will help the client receive some calories, which this client needs. Option #1 is incorrect. It would be unsafe to take the client outdoors. Option #2 is incorrect. The client is unlikely to be able to sit down for a game, and competitive events, such as cards, are inappropriate for a manic client. Option #4 is incorrect. The client believes he is president; the delusion is part of the disease. The client is also unlikely to stay in his room.

5.14 ① Option #1 is the correct answer. It is essential to find out if the client has made statements regarding, or a plan, concerning suicide to prevent a suicide attempt. Options #2, #3, and #4 all can provide

valuable information, but none outweigh the safety concern of suicide.

5.15 ③ Option #3 is the correct answer. This response is empathetic to the client, validates the client's feelings, and also by asking how the client is coping, will help the nurse assess the needs of the client. Option #1 disregards the client's feelings. Option #2 is false reassurance. Option #4, the nurse is discussing a personal event, not the feelings of the client.

5.16 ① Option #1 is the correct answer. The client made a reasonable request, which the nurse should respect. Option #2 is incorrect for that reason. Option #3 is incorrect. That information is not pertinent to the situation. Option #4 is incorrect. The client had a change in living situation, which can be stressful, however, is actively seeking a support system, which is a positive coping skill for alcoholism / drug abuse.

5.17 ② Option #2 is the correct answer. It is essential the nurse determine if the young man has a plan to commit suicide in place. Options #1, #3 and #4 are all opened ended questions that are good for assessment purposes, however, the need to determine suicide risk is paramount to this scenario. Note that options #1, #3, and #4 address feelings, but option #2 addresses safety!

5.18 ② Option #2 is the correct answer. Removing objects from the client's reach is appropriate. An item (such as silverware) could potentially be used by the client to harm themselves, or someone else. The nurse approaches the client in a calm manner, and gives a clear and firm command. The client should be removed from the situation. Option #1 is incorrect. The client should be taken out of the situation, and it would require the agitated client be left alone to remove other clients, which is unsafe. Option #3 is incorrect, as it removes the other clients. A tranquilizer may be indicated, but the nurse should attempt to manage the situation first. Option #4 is inappropriate.

I CAN Publishing®, INC.

5.19 ① Option #1 is the correct answer. The finding of the client on the floor surrounded by the men of the family indicates a planned, thoughtful process. It is essential for the nurse to determine if a ritual or other cultural practice is taking place regarding the death of this client, and respect the practice. Options #2, #3, and #4 are incorrect. Prior to moving the client, the nurse needs to know if that is appropriate. Notifying the supervisor is not appropriate. Option #4 is not justified as the placement of the client and the family members are planned.

5.20 ② Option #2 is the correct answer. This response allows the nurse to explore the client's statement and is an assessment question. The client is asking the nurse for assistance for the family, and in order to respond appropriately, the nurse must determine what the client needs. The nurse needs more information. Option #1 is incorrect. End of life care should involve the family and assist the client and the family transition through the grieving process. (Denial, anger, bargaining, depression, acceptance) Option #3 is incorrect. The nurse should facilitate communication among the family, and encourage the client to communicate with the family instead of communicating on behalf of the client. Option #4 is a correct statement, but the nurse has not determined if the family is in denial, which makes this statement incorrect.

5.21 ② Option #2 is the correct answer. These are all assessment findings that are found in a dying person. Option #1 is incorrect because edema may increase in the dying person. Option #3 is incorrect, as constipation is problematic in the dying client due to decreased fluid intake, immobility, and the use of narcotics. Option #4 is incorrect, as the dying person will not become more alert. The other symptoms listed for options #1, #3, and #4 are correct findings for the dying client.

5.22 ③ Option #3 is the correct answer. This client has clearly suffered a loss in the form of an amputation, and the client must be assisted through the grieving

process. Validating this out loud to the client, along with giving "permission" to grieve the loss is the most therapeutic response. Option #1 disregards the feelings expressed by the client. Option #2 does not recognize the client's feelings of loss or the client individually. Option #4 is incorrect. The client is grieving, which is a normal response to loss, real or perceived. Counseling may be warranted, but the scenario does not indicate the client is not progressing through the grief process, not coping, or desires counseling.

5.23 ② Option #2 is the correct answer. The client has just been informed of a life changing event, and it is normal to "deny" the ramifications of the loss. This is an appropriate short term coping mechanism. (Denial, anger, bargaining, depression, acceptance) Options #1, #3, and #4 are not therapeutic responses in this scenario.

5.24 ④ Option #4 is the correct answer. The nurse is attempting to explore with the family member reasons for feeling the need to stay. A busy shift on a medical surgical unit is a common event. The nurse may have exhibited a hurried manner, failed to return for a follow up assessment, or the client may have expressed a need that was unmet. By asking the family member what their perception of the evening was, the nurse could reassure or explain the situation as needed. Option #1 gives the impression the nurse is overwhelmed and unable to meet the needs of the assigned client. Option #2 is not therapeutic, nor does it assess the concern of the family member. Option #3 is unprofessional and inappropriate.

5.25 ③ Option #3 is the correct answer. It is imperative the nurse notify the physician of the client's request to assure the wishes of the client will be met. Options #1 and #2 disregard the client's request. Option #4 does attempt to make the staff aware, but does not ensure accountability. By notifying the surgeon of the client's request, and documenting the process, the nurse is covering self from liability if this request is not met.

5.26 ① Option #1 is the correct answer. Spiritual and religious practices of client must be respected, and the nurse needs to allow the client time to employ the positive impact of religion / spirituality on health. Options #2 and #3 are not appropriate at this time. The medication is timed; therefore, there is some flexibility in the time it is administered. For example, a medication ordered at 1400 that is administered at 1410 is not clinically significant. If the client can finish the prayer in that time, the nurse should allow the 10 minutes. If the prayer is not completed in a reasonable amount of time, then an interruption/ explanation would be warranted. Option #4 is not correct. If the medication is timed and an alteration needs to be made in scheduling, the appropriate person to notify is the physician, not the pharmacist.

5.27 ③ Option #3 is the correct answer. Option #3 validates the wife's observations and also educates the wife that is essential to care for herself in order to care for her spouse. Option #1 may be true. The client may forget the events that cause the frustration and anger, but this option does not offer any teaching and is only a statement of fact. Option #2 acknowledges that this is normal, but is an assessment in nature, and does not provide any teaching. Option #4 is information that may or may not be true. A diagnosis of dementia does not mandate admission to a care facility, and at this time, there is no teaching involved.

5.28 ② Option #2 is correct. Option #2 validates the difficulty some individuals have with role changes, and asks an open ended question without judgment. Option #1 disregards the finding that the infant is crying, and the new mother is not reacting to this. Option #3 is inappropriate. There is no indication that the father is/is not involved in the life of the woman or infant. This question assesses the relationship between the parents, not the relationship between the infant and the mother. Option #4 is judgmental in nature, and does not validate or assess the situation, as Option #2.

5.29 ③④⑤ Options #3, #4 and #5 are correct. This question is evaluating the NCLEX® activity: "Assess client for drug/alcohol withdrawal." These options include clinical findings for clients experiencing alcohol withdrawal. Additional clinical findings for client may include restlessness, depressed mood, irritability, vital signs are elevated, so the HR would be elevated and the BP would be increased (Options #1 and #2). A late symptom is tactile hallucinations of "bugs crawling" on the skin.

5.30 ① Option #1 is the correct answer. Option #1 is an open ended question that encourages verbalization from the client and assesses if there are changes or other reasons that would cause the anxiety the client is feeling. Option #2 explores issues of depression, however, the mother is complaining of stress, not depression. Option #3 assumes the woman has insight to the cause of the anxiety, and implies that the woman is responsible for generating the feelings without reason. Option #4 is about the nurse, not assisting the client.

5.31 ② Option #2 is the correct answer. Option #2 needs to be evaluated first due to safety issues. Options #1, #3, and #4 are not going to hurt anyone.

5.32 ④ Option #4 is the correct answer. The client has received tragic information, and a common initial reaction to an overwhelming event is denial. This is an effective (short term) coping mechanism that allows the client to protect himself. Option #4 is the most appropriate and therapeutic in this situation. The client is expressing their feelings, which the nurse needs to allow, and the best method to encourage this is to remain silent and let the client direct the conversation. Option #1 is not appropriate at this time. The client is not in a position to understand the disease process at this time, and is not requesting information. Option #2 is not appropriate at this time. Option #3 is not indicated, as denial is a common response.

5.33 ② Option #2 is the correct answer. Option #2 identifies the observations made by the LPN, and explores why the UAP is upset. Option #1 is inappropriate and confrontational. Options #3 and #4 are correct statements, however, do not address the sarcastic statement made by the UAP.

5.34 ③ Option #3 is the correct answer. The client has a history of schizophrenia, and is suffering from a hallucination. The client has also had general anesthesia, which could account for some changes in the client's perception. Having a room near the nurses' station, the client can be observed more carefully, and of the above choices, best promotes safety. Option #1 is not appropriate for this situation. Option #2 does provide continuity and information that the charge nurse needs, but is not as imperative as changing room assignment. Option #4 validates the hallucination and is not appropriate.

5.35 ② Option #2 is the correct answer. The therapeutic nurse/client relationship is a mutual learning and corrective emotional experience. The nurse utilizes self and specified clinical techniques in working with the client to facilitate insight and behavioral change. Options #1, #3 and #4 are incorrect because the nurse is doing this for the client versus focusing on the client's needs which are the primary concern.

NOTES

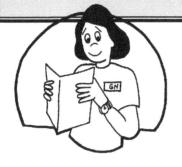

Physiological Integrity
Basic Care and Comfort

*Any fool can make things complex. It takes a touch of a
genius to move in the opposite direction.*
—Albert Einstein

✔ Clarification of this test ...

The minimum standards include providing direct basic care and comfort including
elimination, mobility/immobility, nutrition, non-pharmacological comfort measures,
promoting activities of daily living, complementary and alternative therapies,
promoting client ability to perform activities of daily living, rest / sleep.

- Institute bowel or bladder management
- Perform an irrigation of urinary catheter, bladder, wound, ear, nose, or eye
- Provide for mobility needs (i.e., ambulation, range of motion, transfer to chair, repositioning or the use of adaptive equipment)
- Use measures to maintain or improve client skin integrity
- Provide care to an immobilized client (i.e., traction splint or brace)
- Assist in the care and comfort for a client with a visual and/or hearing impairment
- Use alternative/complementary therapy in providing client care (i.e., music therapy)
- Provide non-pharmacological measures for pain relief (i.e., imagery, massage or repositioning)
- Evaluate pain using a rating scale
- Provide feeding and/or care for client with enteral tubes
- Monitor and provide for nutritional needs of client
- Monitor client intake/output
- Assist with activities of daily living
- Assist in providing postmortem care
- Provide measures to promote sleep/rest

CHAPTER 6: BASIC CARE AND COMFORT

6.1 Which assessment would be most appropriate to report for a client who is taking furosemide (Lasix)?

① Weight on 10/11/12: 110 lbs., weight on 10/12/12:102 lbs.
② Intake and Output: 10/11/12: I–1012 mL, O–1020 mL.
③ Skin turgor elastic.
④ Lips and mucous membranes dry.

6.2 Which of these interventions are appropriate for an older client with a diagnosis of glaucoma to decrease complications of incontinence? *Select all that apply.*

① Reinforce teaching to client on how to perform Kegel exercises daily.
② Review the importance of taking the newly prescribed dicyclomine (Bentyl) as ordered.
③ Review the importance of avoiding or decreasing the intake of caffeine.
④ Discuss the importance of increasing the use of a daily vitamin.
⑤ Review the rationale for avoiding alcohol consumption.

6.3 Which of these statements made by the daughter of an older adult (mother) indicates an understanding of safe skin care for the mother?

① "I will apply sunscreen lotions with a sun protection factor (SPF) of 10 when I take mom out in the sun."
② "I will apply perfumed skin lotions daily to keep mom's skin moist."
③ "I will avoid skin products that contain alcohol."
④ "I will use a strong detergent when washing mom's clothing in order to remove the odors and stains."

6.4 During a teaching session, which of these foods should the nurse include when discussing foods that are good sources of iron. *Select all that apply.*

① Beans
② Dried fruit
③ Spinach
④ Tuna fish
⑤ Yogurt

6.5 What is the priority plan of care for an elderly client with minimal vision who is on a medical unit?

① Softly touch client to let client know the nurse is present.
② When guiding client while walking, walk behind client and place client's hand in the nurse's hand.
③ Assist with meal enjoyment by placing the meal in terms of the face of a clock (i.e., "meat at 6 o'clock").
④ When administering medications, provide client with a full glass of water and explain the number of medications.

6.6 Which of these discharge instructions should be reinforced by the LPN for a client being discharged with Parkinson's disease?

① Advise to purchase a hospital bed for home.
② Discuss the importance of participating in an exercise program during the late afternoon.
③ Install a toilet seat that is raised.
④ Place arms in a dependent position when ambulating.

6.7 The nurse is reviewing the chart of a client who has frequent urinary tract infections. The nurse realizes it is essential to assess the client's:

① Diet
② Weight
③ Normal elimination pattern
④ Temperature

6.8 The UAP says to the LPN, "I am so tired of hearing about bowel movements. Why is it such a big deal to keep track of client's bowel movements?" What response given by the LPN is appropriate?

① "Nurses look at the bowel record and know what to do with the information."
② "No one really pays much attention, but the documentation needs to be done."
③ "It sounds like you are having stress related to work."
④ "The elderly are at high risk for constipation; it is important to keep track, so we can intervene early if need be."

6.9   A client has been diagnosed with peptic ulcer disease. Based on this information, what information should the nurse prepare to discuss with this client?

① Drug therapy
② Stress reduction
③ Nutritional therapy
④ Diagnostic studies

6.10 The LPN is providing AM care to an elderly client who has suffered a severe CVA with hemi-paresis on the right side. Which intervention made by the LPN is most appropriate for a client with a self care deficit?

① Performing AM care as directed by the client.
② Encouraging the client to assist as able.
③ Setting the supplies on the client's right side.
④ Incorporating the assistance of the nursing assistant.

6.11 Which of these nursing actions by the UAP would be a priority of care for a client, during the post-operative period following a thoracic surgery, who is taking enoxaparin (Lovenox) to prevent the development of a DVT or pulmonary embolus?

① Reposition client carefully using the draw sheet.
② Position pillows under knees for comfort when client is in bed.
③ Decrease fluid intake to prevent overload.
④ Report a blood pressure of 120 / 76.

6.12 Which of these plans would be a priority for a client with a C_5 spinal cord injury who is being taught bowel retraining?

① Encourage client to eat a soft diet.
② Decrease fluids and increase fiber intake.
③ Recommend the time for the retraining schedule to be prior to meals.
④ Remain on a routine schedule.

6.13 Which of these plans would be most important for the LPN to implement when preparing to irrigate the ear of a 20-year-old?

① Straighten ear canal by pulling down.
② Forcefully push fluid into the ear canal.
③ Direct water flow toward the bottom of the ear canal.
④ Prepare the irrigating solution to be near body temperature (37 degrees C or approx. 98 degrees F).

6.14 The nurse answers the call light of a client who is requesting to ambulate to the bathroom. The client is quite weak and frail. The nurse determines the client is not on bed rest. How should the LPN proceed?

① Check with the charge nurse.
② Notify the UAP to take the client to the bathroom.
③ Sit the client slowly up on the edge of the bed and have the client sit up and dangle legs prior to getting out of bed.
④ Evaluate all of the vital signs prior to sitting up in bed.

6.15 A client with a history of diarrhea and increased GI motility is started on Bentyl for management of symptoms. What information provided by the LPN will help the client manage the common side effects of this therapy?

① Advise client to decrease oral intake if diarrhea occurs.
② Have hard candy available to manage symptoms of a dry mouth.
③ Take the medication in the morning to avoid nocturia.
④ Take the medication until gone, even if symptoms improve.

6.16 A client has a fever of 101 degrees F, BP–100/62, RR–24/minute, and P–88 beats per minute. The client complains of feeling "awful." How can the nurse assist the client?

① Assess the linens for dampness and wrinkles.
② Offer to assist the client with a cold shower.
③ Notify the charge nurse of the client's complaints.
④ Encourage deep breathing and coughing.

6.17 An adult was riding a bicycle with his son when he hit the curb. As a result, he fell and the LPN found him conscious, alert, but in major pain with a possible left fractured femur. What would be the first nursing action the LPN should implement?

① Assess the dorsalis pedis pulse.
② Assess the circumstances before and after the accident.
③ Request client not to move and immobilize the left leg with a splint.
④ Position client in the Fowler's position.

6.18 The nurse is preparing medications for a client with a feeding tube. After assuring the medications are correct for the client, the nurse crushes them, mixes the medications in water, and goes to the client's bedside, and identifies the client. Which action should the nurse take next?

① Flush the feeding tube.
② Aspirate contents of the feeding tube.
③ Administer the medications.
④ Elevate the head of the bed.

6.19 A client who underwent a TURP is admitted to a post-operative unit, and has continuous bladder irrigation. The client states, "My bladder feels full." The initial action by the nurse is to:

① Palpate the client's bladder.
② Have the client rate pain level on a scale of 1 to 10.
③ Reassure the client this is a normal sensation.
④ Evaluate the catheter for patency.

6.20 A client that has undergone a colectomy yesterday and is running a temperature of 99.4. The client reports a pain level of 6 of 10. What should the LPN do with these findings?

① Notify the physician.
② Notify the charge nurse.
③ Medicate for pain and ambulate the client after medication has been effective.
④ Medicate for pain and turn the client after medication has been effective.

6.21 A mother had a Cesarean delivery, and is complaining of great discomfort with gas and constipation. When this mother notifies the office of the complaints, and speaks to the LPN, the nurse should encourage the client to:

① Increase fluids and ambulation.
② Increase fluids and decrease pain medication.
③ Take an OTC remedy for gas.
④ Reassure the client these findings are normal.

6.22 What would be the priority nursing action for a client receiving a continuous gastric tube feeding at 90 ml per hour who has a residual of 80 ml in the stomach?

① Continue feeding and discard residual.
② Stop feeding and discard residual.
③ Notify physician.
④ Stop the feeding and return to the stomach.

6.23 The home healthcare LPN is visiting a client on hospice. While assessing the client, the nurse finds a hot water bottle on the client's feet. What additional finding would be of greatest concern to the nurse?

① Palpable pedal pulses
② Pain level 4/10
③ Inability to change position independently
④ BP–100/70, RR–20/minute, P–88 beats per minute, T–99.0 degrees F

6.24 A client is to be discharged home using crutches after having surgery on the knee. The client states, "How am I going to get into my apartment? I live on the second floor and there is no elevator." How should the nurse intervene?

① Reassure the client; then review the proper method for crutch use and stairs.
② Notify social services for the need for assistance with the client's living situation.
③ Notify the physician, and request a walker for the client to have after being discharged.
④ Notify the physician the client will not be able to be discharged home due to the current living situation.

6.25 The nurse is observing care being provided by the UAP in a long term care facility. Which behavior by the UAP would indicate a need for further instruction?

① Dressing a client who is capable of dressing themselves with slight assistance.
② Toileting a client when the client requests.
③ Feeding a client thickened fluids who has dysphagia
④ Providing oral care to a client with dentures.

6.26 Which statement made by the client with a left-sided hemiparesis from a CVA indicates an understanding of how to transfer self out of the bed?

① "The wheel chair should be on the right side of the bed."
② "The wheel chair should be on the left side of the bed."
③ "I will use a cane."
④ "I will wait for the physical therapist to lift me out of the bed."

6.27 Nursing care for a client in Buck's traction should include:

① Assessing the site of pain for bleeding or infection.
② Applying topical or antibiotic ointment as ordered.

③ Assessing that the elastic bandages are not too loose or tight.
④ Remove the bandages daily to lubricate the skin.

6.28 Which assessment would be most appropriate for monitoring a client's state of hydration?

① Daily weight.
② I & O.
③ Skin turgor.
④ Characteristics of lips and mucous membranes.

6.29 When evaluating a group of charts for the quality assurance process, which documentation reveals quality care for a group of clients with meningitis who have developed syndrome of inappropriate antidiuretic hormone (SIADH)?

① Clients were encouraged to drink fluids to assist with fluid imbalance.
② Clients were monitored for dilute urine with a specific gravity of 1.001.
③ Clients were weighed daily and HCPs notified if weight increased.
④ Clients were monitored for dry mucous membranes and decrease in skin turgor.

6.30 A client who had an appendectomy is requesting pain medicine post-operative. What assessment would be most appropriate for this client? The nurse questions:

① "What precipitates the pain?"
② "Where is the location of the pain?"
③ "What is the pain sensation?"
④ "On a scale of 0-10, how would you measure your pain?"

6.31 What is the priority of care after the urinary catheter has been removed?

① Encourage client to decrease fluid intake.
② Document size of catheter and client's tolerance of procedure.
③ Evaluate client for normal voiding.
④ Document client teaching.

6.32 Organize these steps in chronological order with #1 being the first step for a client who is having a nasogastric tube removed.

① Assist client into semi-Fowler's position.
② Ask client to hold breath.
③ Assess bowel function by auscultation for peristalsis.
④ Flush tube with 10 ml of normal saline.
⑤ Withdraw the tube gently and steadily.
⑥ Monitor client for nausea and vomiting.

6.33 A geriatric client is admitted to the long term facility with left-sided paralysis. Which clinical data would offer the nurse the most useful information regarding the dietary intake? The client's:

① Favorite foods.
② Ability to chew and swallow.
③ Normal bowel schedule.
④ Routine meal times before admission.

6.34 After a month of taking iron supplements, a client complains of constipation. The nurse should adapt a diet for client to include:

① Oatmeal, green beans, celery.
② Strawberries, rice, mushrooms.
③ Grits, orange juice, cheddar cheese.
④ Past, buttermilk, bananas.

6.35 What is the best way to determine fluid retention for a 7-month-old infant?

① Weigh the infant daily.
② Evaluate abdominal girth weekly.
③ Test the urine for hematuria.
④ Count the number of wet diapers.

I CAN Publishing®, INC.

ANSWERS & RATIONALES

6.1 ① Option #1 is correct. Daily weight is the most appropriate evaluation out of these options. It is the most measurable to evaluate the outcomes. During the last 24 hours there has been a drop of 8 lbs. While options #2, #3 and #4 are correct, they are not a priority to option #1.

 I CAN HINT: Furosemide (Lasix) is prescribed to treat and control edema related to cirrhosis, CHF, renal disease, and hypertension. The "ABCs" will help you remember the clinical findings that must be assessed for when taking this medication include:

Anorexia

BP ↓

Change or drop in weight, **C**ramps–muscle (from ↓ K), **C**alcium ↓

Diarrhea

Electrolytes (↓ K)

Fluid and electrolyte (I & O)

Glucose ↑

Hypotension if lose too much fluid

6.2 ① Options #1, #3, and #5 are correct options.
③ Urinary incontinence is a significant
⑤ contributing factor to falls, fractures, depression, and altered skin integrity, especially in older adult clients. There are six major types of urinary incontinence. These include: stress, urge, overflow, reflex, functional, and total incontinence. Part of the collaborative care for these clients include: teaching how to perform Kegel exercises daily, reviewing the importance of avoiding or decreasing the intake of caffeine, and reviewing the rationale for avoiding alcohol consumption. Specific medications may result in the stimulation of voiding. Vaginal cone therapy may be used to strengthen pelvic muscles for clients with stress incvontinence. Option #2 is incorrect. While dicyclomine (Bentyl) may be used to decrease urgency for a client with a neurogenic or overactive bladder, if the client has a diagnosis of glaucoma and this medication is taken an increase intraocular pressure may occur, so Bentyl should not be administered to this client. The order should be verified due to inappropriateness of this order for a client with glaucoma. Option #4 is incorrect. The vitamin is not prescribed to decrease incontinence.

 I CAN HINT: The key to this question is that the client has glaucoma along with the incontinence. Anticholinergic medications are contraindicated for these clients. The intake of alcohol or caffeine that results in relaxation can cause an increase in the urination. Notice in the stem of the question, if there is a medication, disease, lab value, age, clinical assessment finding, etc., there is a reason, so pay attention. This most likely will be your clue to assist in selecting the correct answer(s).

6.3 ③ Option #3 is correct. Since alcohol is drying to the skin, it should be avoided. Age-related skin changes of the elderly include fragile and dry skin. Option #1 is incorrect since it should have an SPF of 15 or greater to protect against sunburn. Option #2 is incorrect. Skin lotions should be used without perfume since perfume in the lotions may increase skin irritation and increase the risk of injury to the skin resulting in skin breakdown. Option #4 is incorrect. Strong laundry detergents may cause irritation to the skin which can also lead to skin breakdown.

 I CAN HINT: "SKIN" will assist you in recalling priorities for skin care for the elderly client.

Skin—maintain clean, dry skin and wrinkle-free linens. Sun protection factor (SPF) 15 or > when in sun.

Know the importance of repositioning client in bed at least q 2hr. and q1 hr when sitting in chair.

Intake—2,000 to 3,000 mL/day.

Nutrition—meet protein and calorie needs. If serum albumin levels are < 3.5 mg/dL, this is high risk for skin breakdown and may result in a decrease in healing and risk for infection. No lotions with perfume. No strong detergents. No skin products with alcohol.

6.4 ① Options #1, #2, #3 and #4 are correct.
② These are high in iron. Option #5 is not
③ high in iron.
④

6.5 ③ Option #3 is correct. Organizing the meal in a consistent placement will facilitate the client enjoying the foods by knowing where each type of food is located on the plate. A few additional plans that may be helpful for this client with minimal vision may include: indentifying self upon entering the room, always raising side rails for newly sightless persons (i.e., clients wearing postoperative eye patches), walking client around the room and acquainting client with all objects: bed, TV, telephone, etc. Option # 1 is incorrect. The nurse should never touch a client unless client knows nurse is present. Option #2 is incorrect. When guiding client while walking, walk ahead of client and place client's hand in the bend of the nurses' elbow. Option #4 is incorrect. When administering medications, inform client of number of pills; however, what makes this option incorrect is that only a half glass of water should be given in order to avoid spills.

I CAN HINT: Remember for the option to be correct, the entire information must be correct. If part of the option is wrong, the entire option cannot be used as an answer.

6.6 ③ Option #3 is correct. This will help the client remain independent. Option #1 is not necessary for this client since there is no assessment finding mandating this action. Option #2 is the incorrect time

for exercise. It should be planned for late morning when energy is highest and there will be no need to hurry. Option #4 should read for client to swing arms to facilitate balance when ambulating.

6.7 ③ Option #3 is correct. This will assist the nurse in understanding the typical pattern of elimination for this client to better assist with the plan of action. Options #1, #2, and #4 are incorrect for this client. While option #4 is an important assessment for this client, it does not indicate the reason for so many infections. The temperature is a result of the infection not the cause.

6.8 ④ Option #4 is the correct answer. This response provides teaching to the UAP and defines the risk of constipation in the elderly. Option #1 dismisses the request for information from the UAP. Option #2 is a false statement. Option #3 is an open ended question that would encourage the assistant to explore / express feelings of stress; however, the UAP makes a clear request for information.

6.9 ② Option #2 is the correct answer. Option #2 is within the scope of practice for the LPN and a common characteristic of clients suffering from peptic ulcer disease is stress. Options #1, #3, and #4 are the responsibility of the physician/pharmacist /nutritionist. The role of the nurse is to introduce or reinforce information regarding these topics.

6.10 ② Option #2 is correct. Encouraging client to assist as able is most useful for this situation. Option #1 is incorrect since the client may not be able to direct due to client's condition. Option #3 is incorrect since they should be on the opposite side. Option #4 is incorrect since this does not include the focus of the client to assist to demonstrate client's ability.

6.11 ① Option #1 is correct This option provides the safest way to reposition the client who is taking enoxaparin (Lovenox) which is an anticoagulant that can result in bleeding in the extremity if not supported appropriately during repositioning. The draw sheet will facilitate this and prevent skin breakdown. Option #2 is incorrect since this will allow for blood to pool behind the knee and result in further complications with DVTs. Option #3 is incorrect since fluid is necessary to prevent further complications with stasis of blood. Option #4 is incorrect.

6.12 ④ Option #4 is correct. The key to successful bowel and bladder training is consistency with the schedule. The routine schedule is the key to success with this process. Option #1 is incorrect. Option #2 is incorrect. Fluids are always an important part of this process. Option #3 is incorrect. It most likely will be after meals, but the key is consistentcy.

6.13 ④ Option #4 is correct. This is the correct temperature for ear irrigation. If it is too hot or too cold, it can result in dizziness and nausea. Option #1 is incorrect. The correct procedure is to straighten the ear canal by pulling the outer ear up for adults or down for children under 3. Option #2 is incorrect. Fluid should never be forcefully pushed into the ear canal, as this may rupture the eardrum. If nausea, vomiting, or dizziness develop, stop the irrigation immediately. Option #3 is incorrect. The direct water flow should be toward the top of the ear canal to create a circular motion.

6.14 ③ Option #3 is the correct answer. This will assist with orthostatic hypotension and minimize the risk for falls. Option #1 is incorrect since the LPN is able to do ongoing assessments and interventions. Option #2 is incorrect due to the need for an understanding of the risk for falls since the client is weak, frail, and safety issues regarding potential changes in blood pressure. Option #4 is not necessary and is inappropriate when needing to go to the bathroom. Temperature is part of vital signs and is irrelevant to this situation.

6.15 ② Option #2 is correct since this is an anticholinergic medication and can cause a dry mouth. Option #1 is incorrect since diarrhea is not a common side effect. Constipation is a common side effect, so

fluid intake would be appropriate versus decreasing intake. Option #3 is incorrect since a common side effect would not be nocturia but a decrease in urine output (oliguria). Option #4 does not address the question regarding the side effects.

6.16 ① Option #1 is the correct answer. When anyone suffers from a fever it is common to feel "awful". Comfort measures, such as a dry unwrinkled bed, or lip ointment for someone with dry lips go a long way towards recovery. Option #2 is incorrect. A tepid shower/bath may be appropriate for a febrile client, but a cold shower is not. Option #3 may be warranted if the client's condition changes, but based on the information provided; the client suffers from a fever only. Option #4 is incorrect. The client is complaining of discomfort. If the client was on bedrest or post-operative, this intervention would be correct, but that is not the case based on the information provided.

6.17 ③ Option #3 is correct. The priority is to provide safety and prevent further damage to leg. Options #1 and #2 involve assessment finding. Option #4 is not necessary for this client. The client is not in respiratory distress.

6.18 ④ Option #4 is the correct answer. The nurse must elevate the head of the bed in order to prevent aspiration before, during, and 30 minutes after administration of any fluids via a feeding tube. Options #1, #2, and #3 are incorrect, and do not protect the client from the risk of aspiration.

6.19 ④ Option #4 is the correct answer. When a client is receiving continuous irrigation and complains of bladder fullness, it is imperative to evaluate the drainage bag and make sure there are no occlusions and that urine is freely draining. Option #1 is incorrect. The client should not have a full bladder, and assessing for bladder distension is not the appropriate initial intervention. Option #2 deals with the sensation of pain versus feeling a full bladder. Option #3 is an incorrect statement.

6.20 ③ Option #3 is the correct answer. A client that is in pain and running a low grade temperature is at risk for atelectasis, and it is appropriate to employ interventions to clear the lungs of secretions; the best method to do this is with ambulation. Option #1 and #2 may be appropriate if the LPN's interventions fail. Option #4 is acceptable; turning the client will help improve respiratory function, but is not better than ambulation

Adverse effects of immobility: **AWFUL** = Atelectasis, Wasting of bones, Functional loss of muscle, Urinary stasis, Last but not least, constipation

6.21 ① Option #1 is the correct answer. An increase in fluid intake and ambulation may be enough to solve the mother's symptoms. Option #2 is incorrect. Although pain medications are constipating in nature, this woman has had serious surgery, and will not function well without adequate pain control. Option #3 is not as effective as ambulation in decreasing gas. Option #4 is incorrect. These may be common findings, but are not considered "normal".

Adverse effects of immobility: **AWFUL** = Atelectasis, Wasting of bones, Functional loss of muscle, Urinary stasis, Last but not least, constipation

6.22 ④ Option #4 is correct. Residuals less than 150 ml should be returned due to risk of altering fluid and electrolytes. Stop feeding if residual is over 50% of the volume client gets in 1 hour. Option #1 is incorrect. Discarding residual is not correct. Option #2 is incorrect as well. Option #3 does not address the issue first.

6.23 ③ Option #3 is the correct answer. It is imperative the nurse determine if the client has the ability to move away from a heat source, such as a hot water bottle, in order to prevent injury. A heat device should never be applied to a client with an altered mental status, or the inability to move away from the source of heat. Option #1 is normal. Option #2 is of concern, but does not outweigh the safety issue presented. Option #4, while the blood pressure may be low, the pulse and respirations are WNL.

6.24 ① Option #1 is the correct answer. Clients can safely navigate stairs. Option #2, #3 and #4 are inappropriate for this situation.

CRUTCH WALKING: Good goes to heaven (*up the stairs, lead with good leg*), Bad goes to hell (*down the stairs, lead with bad leg*) (*Nursing Made Insanely Easy,* Rayfield & Manning)

6.25 ① Option #1 is the correct answer. The UAP needs to promote the abilities of the client, and by doing things the client is capable of doing themselves, the client is at risk to lose this ability. Options #2, #3, and #4 are appropriate and do not require further teaching.

6.26 ① Option #1 is the correct answer. When teaching paralyzed clients how to transfer themselves, it is important for them to understand the strong side leads. Options #2, #3, #4 are ineffective.

6.27 ③ Option #3 is the correct answer. Assessment is needed to make sure circulation is not being compromised. Option #1 is incorrect because Buck's traction is a type of skin traction. There are no pins. Option #2 is incorrect because skin traction has no need for topical ointment. Option #4 is incorrect because the skin is not lubricated under the bandage.

6.28 ① Option #1 is correct. Daily weight is the most appropriate evaluation out of these options. It is the most measurable. While Options #2, #3, and #4 are correct, they are not a priority to option #1.

6.29 ③ Option #3 is correct. SIADH has too much antidiuretic hormone which results in fluid retention. Weight increase should be reported. Option #1 is incorrect. Fluid should be restricted. Option #2 is incorrect. Specific gravity would be high. Option #4 would be appropriate for Diabetes Insipidus.

6.30 ④ Option #4 is correct. This option evaluates the pain based on the appropriate Standard of Practice. The other options are not as measurable as #4.

6.31 ③ Option #3 is correct. Client should be voiding normally within 24 hours. Options #1, #2, and #4 are incorrect. Option #1 should be increased versus decreased. Option #2 is not totally correct. The size of the catheter should have been documented when it was placed. Option #4 is important, but is not a priority for this question.

6.32 ③ Option #3 is the first step. Option #1 is
① the second step. Option #4 is the third
④ step. Flushing will ensure that the tube
② doesn't contain stomach contents that
⑤ could irritate tissues during tube removal.
⑥ Option #2 is the fourth step. This is to close epiglottis. Option #5 is the fifth step. Option #6 is the sixth step. For 48 hours, monitor client for GI dysfunction including nausea, vomiting, abdominal distention, and food intolerance.

6.33 ② Option #2 is correct. The ability of the client to chew and swallow will be the basis of planning. Options #1 and #4 will not make any difference if he cannot chew. Option #3 would be important in avoiding constipation, but does not answer question regarding dietary intake.

6.34 ① Option #1 is correct. This option contains foods highest in fiber to assist in counteracting constipation. The other options do not have as high a fiber content.

6.35 ① Option #1 is correct. Fluid retention is best detected by weighing daily and noting a gaining trend. Options #2 and #3 are incorrect and will not provide information regarding fluid retention. Option #4 can provide an estimation of the amount of urine output but not about fluid retention.

NOTES

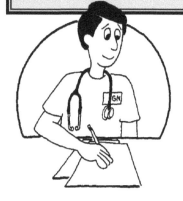

CHAPTER 7

Physiological Integrity
Pharmacological Therapies

Words are of course the most powerful
DRUG used by mankind.
—Unknown

✔ Clarification of this test ...

Clarification of this test includes performing and directing activities necessary for safe administration of medications (adverse effects, blood and blood products, pharmacological interactions, pain management, and TPN). Pharmacology is one of the heaviest weighted sections of the NCLEX® exam.

- ☞ Perform calculations needed for medication administration

- ☞ Reinforce education to client regarding medications

- ☞ Evaluate client response to medication (i.e., adverse reactions, interactions, therapeutic effects)

- ☞ Follow the rights of medication administration

- ☞ Maintain medication safety practices (i.e., storage, checking for expiration dates, and compatibility)

- ☞ Reconcile and maintain medication list or medication administration record (i.e., prescribed medications, herbal supplements, over-the-counter medications)

- ☞ Collect required data prior to medication administration

- ☞ Administer medication by oral route

- ☞ Administer intravenous piggyback (secondary) medications

- ☞ Administer medication by gastrointestinal tube (i.e., g-tube, nasogastric (NG) tube, g-button, or j-tube)

- ☞ Administer a subcutaneous, intradermal, or intramuscular medication

- ☞ Administer medication by ear, eye, nose, inhalation, rectum, vagina, or skin route

- ☞ Count narcotics/controlled substances

- ☞ Calculate and monitor intravenous (IV) flow rate

- ☞ Monitor transfusion of blood product

- ☞ Administer pharmacological pain medication

- ☞ Maintain pain control devices (i.e., epidural, patient control analgesia, peripheral nerve catheter)

7.1   A client has taken levothyroxine sodium (Synthroid) 0.4 mg daily for 4 days. Which symptoms suggest that the nurse should recommend a change in the client's medication?

① Nervousness and difficulty sleeping
② Tired with no energy
③ Coarse hair and skin
④ Persistent weight gain

7.2   Which one of these clients should be seen initially after shift report?

① A client with an order for interferon 2A (Roferon-A), but the RN refuses to administer due to client's history of egg allergy.
② A client who is receiving doxorubicin (Adriamycin) and complaining of nausea and vomiting.
③ A client with cancer who is receiving vincristine (Oncovin) and is complaining of discomfort at IV site.
④ A client with cancer who is receiving bleomycin (Blenoxane) and is beginning to present with alopecia.

7.3   Which of these clinical observations should the UAP report to the nurse for a client with a brain tumor who is taking dexamethasone (Decadron)? *Select all that apply.*

① Weight gain of 3 lbs. since yesterday.
② Tremors and diaphoretic skin.
③ Blood pressure change from 150/90 to 120/78
④ Complaints of a sore throat.
⑤ Moist cough.

7.4   What would be most important to monitor for a client with a spinal cord injury who is taking naproxen (Aleve) and dexamethasone (Decadron)?

① Decrease in daily weight.
② Hemoglobin and Hematocrit.
③ Muscle cramps in legs.
④ Signs of hypoglycemia.

7.5   Which of these actions by the client who is using a metered-dose inhaler (MDI) for taking albuterol (Proventil) indicates an appropriate understanding for the use of this MDI? *Select all that apply.*

① When two puffs are needed, client allows for 1 minute elapse between the two.
② The activation of the MDI is coordinated with expiration.
③ Special care is taken to not shake the inhaler prior to using.
④ When using the MDI, the client inspires slowly.
⑤ Client understands that albuterol (Proventil) is used on a continuous basis in the absence of symptoms.

7.6   Which instruction should be reinforced by the LPN to a client taking tetracycline HCL?

① Take with a glass of milk during meals.
② Recommend taking with a small amount of water.
③ Recommend taking an antacid with the medication to prevent an ulcer.
④ Avoid exposure to direct sunlight.

7.7   A client calls the physician's office with the complaint of nausea, vomiting and diarrhea for the past two days. The nurse advises the client to eat a bland diet, increase fluids, and to rest. Which of these medications would be of greatest concern to the nurse? A client who is taking:

① Warfarin (Coumadin).
② Clarithromycin (Biaxin).
③ Lithium.
④ Atenolol (Tenormin).

7.8   What teaching information should the nurse provide to the elderly client who has an order to begin taking risperidone (Risperdal)?

① "Wear dark glasses during the day, and report an increase in anxiety immediately."
② "Increase fluid intake and change positions slowly."
③ "Report constipation and signs of infection immediately."
④ "This medication should be taken until it is gone regardless of symptoms."

7.9 A client comes to the office reporting anxiety. The physician orders Xanax 0.5-1mg orally three times daily. Which of these clients would require the nurse to question the order?

① a 36-year-old woman who has a history of depression
② a 54-year-old man who has had heart surgery
③ a 74-year-old with hypertension
④ a 58-year-old with a history of alcoholism

7.10 A client is started on tranylcypromine (Parnate) therapy. Which statement made by the client indicates an understanding of the side effects of Parnate?

① "I do not need to change my diet."
② "I should avoid aged cheese and wine."
③ "I should avoid foods high in vitamin K."
④ "I should increase my fluid intake."

7.11 The LPN is reinforcing the teaching for a client in an assisted living facility about what not to take with verapamil (Calan). What response by the client indicates an understanding of this plan?

① "I will not drink cranberry juice in the morning with my medication."
② "I will not drink milk with my dinner."
③ "I will not drink grapefruit juice in the morning with my medication."
④ "I will take my vitamin D in the morning with my breakfast."

7.12 Which of these clinical assessment findings would indicate a desired outcome for a client taking lansoprazole (Prevacid) who is on a mechanical ventilator?

① Client will be able to sleep between nursing care.
② Client will experience no symptoms of infection.
③ Client will experience an increase in the quality of respirations.
④ Client will experience relief of any gastrointestinal symptoms.

7.13 An elderly neighbor approaches the nurse and says, "I found at the grocery store today a supplement that is guaranteed to help with my vision. I can't wait to start taking it." What response should the nurse make?

① "That is great, what is it called?"
② "Are you taking other medications or supplements?"
③ "That was probably a waste of money."
④ "What kind of problems are you having with your vision?"

7.14 The client reports taking Pseudoephedrine (Sudafed) for treatment of congestion. The client is also taking tranylcypromine (Parnate). What would be the priority nursing plan?

① Monitor blood pressure.
② Monitor Intake and Output.
③ Monitor mood changes.
④ Monitor for bradycardia.

7.15 Which clinical finding would be most important for the LPN to report for a client who is receiving Diltiazem (Cardizem)?

① Heart rate dropped from 72 to 60 beats per minute.
② Most recent potassium level – 3.5 mEq/L.
③ Blood pressure 108/74.
④ Most recent digoxin (Lanoxin) level– 1.2 ng/ml.

7.16 Which of these orders should the nurse question administering?

① Meloxicam (Mobic) to a client with osteoarthritis.
② Naproxen (Naprosyn) to a client with general aches with a history of a gastric ulcer.
③ Psyllium (Metamucil) to an elderly client with chronic constipation.
④ Rantidine (Zantac) to a client with a duodenal ulcer.

7.17 What is the earliest sign and symptom of digitalis toxicity for an eighty-year-old client?

    ① Acute confusion.
    ② Heart Rate–58 BPM.
    ③ Muscle cramps.
    ④ Yellow vision.

7.18 A client has an order to administer furosemide (Lasix) po at 9 PM daily. What is the appropriate nursing action at this time for this client?

    ① Assess the heart rate prior to administering the medication.
    ② Evaluate the vital signs prior to administering the medication.
    ③ Notify the provider of care and question the time for administering the drug.
    ④ Review the sodium and potassium level prior to administering.

7.19 Which medication should the nurse administer first?

    ① Lantus insulin for a client with a serum glucose level of 190 mg/dL.
    ② Nifedipine (Procardia) for a client with hypertension.
    ③ Meperidine (Demerol) for a client with a headache rated a 7.
    ④ Psyllium (Metamucil) for a client with chronic constipation.

7.20 The nurse should instruct the client to take pravastatin (Pravachol):

    ① With a low-fat lunch.
    ② 30 minutes before breakfast.
    ③ Between lunch and dinner.
    ④ At bedtime with a snack.

7.21 After receiving a repeat dose of albuterol (Ventolin) per nebulizer, the client states, "I feel as if my heart is racing." What would be the appropriate response from the LPN?

    ① Place client immediately on monitor and perform a chest x-ray.
    ② Reassure client this is a common side effect from this drug.
    ③ Immediately notify the provider of care.
    ④ Place client on oxygen at 4 L.

7.22 What is the priority of care for a client who has an order for Regular Insulin 8 IU Subcutaneous in A.M.?

    ① Verify client identity prior to administering.
    ② Transcribe to appropriate document.
    ③ Notify provider of care and request a revised order.
    ④ Evaluate serum glucose prior to administration.

7.23 Which of these clients should the LPN question administering the medication?

    ① The client receiving warfarin (Coumadin) with a pT of 90 seconds (control–15 seconds).
    ② The client receiving Digoxin with an apical heart rate of 62 BPM.
    ③ The client receiving Lisinopril (Zestril) with a potassium level of 3. 7 mEq/L.
    ④ The client receiving nitroglycerin with a blood pressure of 140/80.

7.24 Which teaching should be reinforced by the LPN after the RN initiates the teaching plan for a client who has an order for an oral iron supplement?

    ① Advise the client to take the iron with milk.
    ② Recommend taking the medication at night.
    ③ Discuss that the stools may be greenish black.
    ④ Review the importance of crushing the tablets.

7.25 A geriatric client is receiving epoetin alfa (Epogen) for chronic renal failure. While reviewing lab results, which of these would indicate a therapeutic effect?

    ① Hematocrit of 48%.
    ② Hemoglobin 10 g/dL.
    ③ WBC of 8000 / mm^3.
    ④ Platelet count 390,000 cells / mm^3.

7.26 An LPN is caring for a 70-year-old client who is taking docusate sodium (Colace). Which of these clinical assessment findings would indicate an undesirable effect from this medication?

① Orange urine
② Abdominal distention with absent bowel sounds
③ HR of 72 beats per minute
④ Abdominal cramps

7.27 Which statement made by the client indicates a correct understanding of the Pneumococcal vaccines?

① "I'm so glad that this vaccine will prevent me from getting pneumonia again."
② "I know I need to get the pneumococcal vaccine for my 4-year-old son since he gets recurrent ear infections and attends a day care center."
③ "I needed a pneumococcal vaccine since I have COPD even if I am only 60."
④ "I need to get a pneumococcal shot every 10 years after I am 65."

7.28 Which statement made by the client indicates a need for further teaching about the inactivated influenza vaccine?

① "I may get this vaccination even though I am allergic to eggs."
② "I do not need this vaccination since it is June."
③ "I know that this vaccination can cause fatigue and muscle aches."
④ "I should get this vaccination since I am HIV positive."

7.29 A client has an order for Humulin N 70/30 insulin 18 units every morning subcutaneously plus the following sliding scale for Humulin Regular U-100 insulin before meals and at bedtime subcutaneously.

Blood Glucose Level	
(mg/dL)	Regular Insulin
Less than 70 mg/dL	Call MD
70-120 mg/dL	0 units
121-175 mg/dL	2 units
176-225 mg/dL	4 units
226-275 mg/dL	6 units
276-325 mg/dL	8 units
325-375 mg/dL	10 units
376-425 mg/dL	12 units
Greater than 426 mg/dL	Call MD

At 0800, the client's blood sugar is 384 milligram/deciliters. Shade in the amount the nurse will administer.

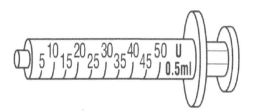

7.30 The client with hypothyroidism (myxedema) is taking levothyroxine (Synthroid) daily and notes such an improvement in the way he feels that he doubles the dose. Which of these clinical findings should be reported to the healthcare provider?

① Blood pressure 100/75
② Pulse 105
③ Urine output of 175–220 mLs every 3 to 4 hours
④ Weight gain of 3 pounds

7.31 While assessing the diabetic education, the nurse concludes that the client with type I diabetes mellitus who takes glipizide (Glucotrol) needs further education when which statement is made?

① "Need to eat six small meals daily to maintain an even sugar level."
② "Should always have some hard candy to use if my sugar is low."
③ "Usually skip breakfast because I don't take the time to eat."
④ "Will purchase medical identification jewelry to wear at all times."

7.32 A client taking prednisone for rheumatoid arthritis now has pitting edema of both legs. What is the nurse's best first action?

① Assess the client's pulse, blood pressure, and breath sounds.
② Document the finding and notify the physician immediately.
③ Instruct the client to sit with legs elevated at every chance.
④ Teach the client to weigh herself daily and keep a diary.

7.33 The nurse assesses the need for further education for the client with rheumatoid arthritis who is taking celecoxib (Celebrex) when the following statement is made:

① "I could have renal failure while taking this medication."
② "Might be at risk for a stroke."
③ "Should not take aspirin when I am taking Celebrex."
④ "Will not have problems with stomach bleeding."

7.34 The nurse instructs a client with diverticulitis who is being treated with psyllium (Metamucil) to take the medication:

① By chewing the granules.
② Immediately after mixing.
③ In the morning and at bedtime.
④ On an empty stomach.

7.35 Which nursing considerations must be incorporated for the geriatric population while taking acetazolamide (Diamox)?

① Observe for a decrease in incontinence.
② Discontinue Diamox abruptly.
③ The elderly may be more sensitive to diuretic-induced hypotension and electrolyte imbalances.
④ Start the elderly on the full recommended dose; decrease dose if needed.

ANSWERS & RATIONALES

7.1 ① Nervousness and insomnia suggest an overdose of thyroid hormone replacement therapy. Options #2, #3, and #4 are symptoms of hypothyroidism—the reason for giving this medication.

 I CAN HINT: In *Pharmacology Made Insanely Easy*, there is a great image of "Morbid Matilda" who is taking Synthroid. We named her this, so you could remember she may have myxedema. Great nickname for her is M &M's. (Matilda Myxedema) "THROID" will assist you in remembering the major care for this drug.

TSH, T$_3$, T$_4$–Monitor

Hypo/Hyperthyroidism must be monitored

Review with client how to take pulse and report if > 100 bpm

Observe clinical improvement in 3 to 4 days

Increase metabolic rate–action

Do NOT change brands of drug

7.2 ③ Option #3 is correct. Vincristine (Oncovin) is a vesicant and can be very damaging to the tissue. If client is complaining of discomfort at the site, the nurse needs to go and assess client immediately. Many times there will be a protocol for administration of antidotes and application of heat or cold prior to administering this drug. Option #1 is good practice since interferon is grown in eggs, and if there is an allergy there is a risk for the client to develop a hypersensitivity reaction. This is a good practice not to administer, and notify healthcare provider. Options #2 and #4 are expected outcomes, so would not be a priority over option #4.

I CAN HINT: An easy way to remember the undesirable effect with vincristine (Oncovin) is to remember the "**Vs**". Vesicants damage the veins Very much if extraVasation occurs. These drugs include Vincristine, Vinblastine, and Vinorelbine. When you see a question on these with a focus on discomfort at the IV site, you can safely know that this is a priority due to the damage that can occur.

7.3 ① Options # 1, #4, and #5 are correct.
④ Dexamethasone (Decadron) is a
⑤ corticosteroid. It is an anti-inflammatory and can result in an increase in fluid retention as indicated by Option #1, weight gain and may result in Option #5, the moist cough. Option #4 is correct since the medication may cause the client to be immunosuppressed. The client may present with an infection such as the sore throat as many of the other signs of infection may be masked. Option #2 is incorrect. These symptoms indicate a complication with hypoglycemia and the actual undesirable effect of this medication would be hyperglycemia. *Remember that "if the skin is hot and dry the blood sugar is high, but cool and clammy means they need some candy."* Option #3 is incorrect since the BP has decreased. The undesirable effect from this medication would be an elevation in the blood pressure.

I CAN HINT: An understanding of the drug dexamethasone (Decadron) is the key for answering this question correctly! "CUSHING" will assist you in organizing the key facts for this corticosteroid. This will assist you with any drug in this category.

Cushing-like symptoms

b**U**ffalo hump

Sodium ↑, sweating

Hyperglycemia

Increased in BP, appetite, immunocompromised

Not healing quickly

GI upset

Some **P**eople **G**et **C**old = Remember there is a **U** in C**U**shing, so start with the arrow going ↑ (**U**p)

Sodium ↑

Potassium ↓

Glucose ↑

Calcium ↓

7.4 ② Option #2 is correct. Both of these drugs can cause GI irritation which can result in peptic ulcers that can cause bleeding. Monitoring the hemoglobin and hematocrit will assist the nurse in determining if the client is developing any complications from bleeding. Option #1 is incorrect; although the dexamethasone (Decadron) may result in fluid retention, naproxen (Aleve) would not contribute to this clinical finding. The focus of the question is for both of these drugs. Option #3 could be an issue with dexamethasone (Decadron) alone, but not with naproxen (Aleve). Option #4 is incorrect since the concern would be more with hyperglycemia, but still not an issue for naproxen (Aleve).

I CAN HINT: The key to answering this question appropriately is to remember the common undesirable effects both medications have in common. The book, *Pharmacology Made Insanely Easy* by Manning and Rayfield has great images to help this information stick in the long term memory. One look at *"Cushy Carl"* and you will remember forever the major undesirable effects from dexamethasone (Decadron).

7.5 ① ④ Option #1 and #4 are correct. Option #2 is incorrect since this is coordinated with inspiration. Option #3 is incorrect since the inhaler should be shaken up prior to use to provide an adequate amount of inhalation medication. Option #5 is incorrect. Albuterol (Proventil) is used for short-term relief of acute reversible airway problems. This is not used on a continuous basis in absence of symptoms.

I CAN HINT: "INHALERS" will assist you in organizing the sequence of events for clients taking meds with a metered-dose inhaler (MDI).

Inhaler cap removed; wash hands

Note to shake 5-6 times

Hold inhaler with mouthpiece at bottom

And hold the inhaler with thumb near the mouthpiece + index and middle fingers at top

Locate inhaler approximately 2 to 4 cm (1-2 in) away from front of mouth

Encourage to take a DB and hold for 5–10 seconds and then exhale

Reposition head back slightly + press the inhaler. As the client presses the inhaler, begin a slow, deep breath that lasts for 3–5 sec. facilitating delivery to air passages. When two puffs are needed, allow for 1 minute between the two.

Slowly hold breath for 10 sec. to allow the med. to deposit in airways. After taking inhaler out of mouth, slowly exhale through nose and pursed lips. Resume normal breathing.

7.6 ④ Option #4 is the correct answer. Clients who take Tetracycline HCl have an increase risk of developing photosensitivity, and this may persist for some time after the drug has been discontinued. Option #1 is incorrect since milk may counteract the effectiveness of the medication by altering the absorption. It is recommended that it should also be taken on an empty stomach. Option #2 is incorrect since the client should take this with a full glass of water. Option #3 is incorrect since an antacid may alter the absorption of the medication.

I CAN HINT: Refer to *Pharmacology Made Insanely Easy*, by Manning & Rayfield. "STOP" Sunlight sensitivity, Take with a full glass of water, Omit antacid, iron, milk, Put drug into empty stomach.

7.7 ③ Option #3 is the correct answer. Since Lithium is a salt and the client is losing fluid and electrolytes from the nausea, vomiting, and diarrhea, there is a risk for dehydration with the risk of developing Lithium toxicity. Options #1, #2, and #4 are incorrect, as there is not a possibility of toxicity. A client receiving warfarin (Coumadin), Biaxin, or Tenormin should be in therapeutic range. A client who is receiving lithium therapy has a narrow range 0.6-1.2 (magic 2's in the *Nursing Made Insanely Easy* book will help you remember drug values), and with dehydration there is a high risk for toxicity.

I CAN HINT: LITHIUM = Levels, Incontinence, Thirst/Thyroid, Hand tremors, Increase fluids, Unsteady, Manic/ Morton's salt (*Pharmacology Made Insanely Easy*, Manning & Rayfield)

7.8 ② Option #2 is the correct answer. Risperidone (Risperdal) is an antipsychotic medication, which has many side effects. Option #1 is incorrect. Sunlight sensitivity can occur, however, anxiety levels should not increase, in fact, sedation and sleepiness are common. Option #3 is incorrect as constipation is commonly due to the anticholinergic effects of these medications, therefore, there is no need to report this to the physician. Signs of infection should be reported. Option #4 is incorrect. These instructions are essential with antibiotic therapy, not antipsychotic drugs.

I CAN HINT: STANCE = Sedation/ sunlight sensitivity, Tardive dyskinesia, Anticholinergic/agranulocytosis, Neuroleptic malignant syndrome, Cardiac arrhythmias (orthostatic hypotension), Extrapyramidal (akathesia) (*Pharmacology Made Insanely Easy*, Manning & Rayfield)

7.9 ④ Option #4 is the correct answer. There are no immediate contraindications for Options #1, #2, or #3. Option #4 is of greatest concern as this client has a known history of abuse, and is at greatest risk to abuse a benzodiazepine.

I CAN HINT: BATS = Beta adrenergic blockers/benzodiazepines, Antihistamines, Tricyclics, SSRI's

7.10 ② Option #2 is the correct answer. Tranylcypromine (Parnate) is a MAO inhibitor. These medications require dietary changes be made in order to avoid any foods or medications that are high in tyramine. If this medication is taken with tyramine, this could result in a hypertensive crisis. Option #1 is incorrect for this reason. Option #3 is the indication for a client on Coumadin. Option #4 is not indicated for Monoamine Oxidase Inhibitors. (*Pharmacology Made Insanely Easy*, Manning & Rayfield)

7.11 ③ Option #3 is the correct answer. Grapefruit juice may increase the serum levels and effect when used with Calcium Channel Blockers. Option #1 has no effect on this drug. Option #2 is fine to take this with milk. Option #4 is incorrect. Clients need to be taught that the effectiveness of the medication may be reduced with the co-administration of vitamin D products.

I CAN HINT: Refer to "Do Not Give a Flip Pill" for further ways to remember testing facts for Calcium Channel Blockers in the (*Pharmacology Made Insanely Easy*, Manning & Rayfield)

7.12 ④ Option #4 is the correct answer. Lansoprazole (Prevacid) is a proton pump inhibitor and suppresses the final step in gastric acid production by forming a covalent bond to two sites of the H+, K+ - ATPase enzyme system at the surface of the gastric parietal cell. This results in an increase in the gastric pH, reducing gastric acid production. Options #1, #2, and #3 are incorrect for this medication.

I CAN HINT: The 7 rights to medication administration: Right route, Right client, Right drug, Right rationale, Right dose, Right time, and Right documentation

7.13 ② Option #2 is the correct answer. Due to the fact that the neighbor is elderly, it is likely that the neighbor takes a medication. The nurse needs to evaluate this in order to protect the possibility of drug/supplement interactions. If the client starts the medication, the nurse should advise the neighbor to consult the physician/pharmacy prior to taking any new supplements. Options #1 and #3 are incorrect. Option #4 is an open ended question that explores the reason the client sought out the treatment, but does not deal with the immediate safety concern.

I CAN HINT: Growth and development throughout the life span.

I CAN HINT: SPINE = Stress management/ safety, Physical activity, Interpersonal relationships, Nutrition, Environmental

7.14 ① Option #1 is the correct answer. Sudafed, an over-the-counter, cold medicine can cause a hypertensive crisis in a client taking a MAO inhibitor. Options #2, #3, and #4 are not correct for these 2 medications.

> **I CAN HINT:** (Refer to MAOI, The "Tyrant" King, in *Pharmacology Made Insanely Easy*, Manning & Rayfield)

7.15 ① Option #1 is the correct answer. Cardizen is a calcium channel blocker that can cause bradycardia. The decrease in the heart rate is the most important parameter to report out of these options. Options #2 and #4 are within normal ranges. Option #3 is not a problem based on the given information.

> **I CAN HINT:** Refer to "Do Not Give a Flip Pill" for further ways to remember testing facts for Calcium Channel Blockers in *Pharmacology Made Insanely Easy*, Manning & Rayfield)

7.16 ② Option #2 should not be administered due to the gastric ulcer; so it is important to question the order. If this medication, however, is prescribed, it should be taken with food to decrease the risk of developing any gastric distress. Option #1 (Mobic) is a nonsteroidal anti-inflammatory drug that is used for clients with osteoarthritis. It decreases pain and inflammation. There is no reason for this order to be questioned. Option #3 is appropriate for clients with chronic constipation. Psyllium (Metamucil) is a bulk-forming laxative, so there is no need to question this order. Option #4 is correct for this client since it reduces gastric acid secretions and does not need to be questioned.

7.17 ① Option #1 is the correct answer. Acute confusion is one of the earliest symptoms of toxicity for the elderly client. This is a different sign and symptom than if the client was 40. Clients can also present with anorexia and / or nausea and vomiting. Option #2 is not a priority over option #1. Bradycardia may definitely be an undesirable effect, and it is imperative to assess the heart rate prior to administering the drug, but it is not the earliest assessment finding indicating a complication with toxicity. Options #3 and #4 are also undesirable effects; they are just not the earliest.

7.18 ③ Option #3 is correct since Lasix is a diuretic and should not be given routinely prior to going to bed. This question is evaluating the knowledge of the right time to administer the diuretic. The rights of medication administration are a priority in preparing meds, and then the nurse proceeds to all of the appropriate assessments. Option #1 is not a priority to #3. Option #2 is similar to #1, but does not address the inappropriate time for administration. Option #4 is very important, but would be done after the nurse had a correct order which would include the correct time.

> **I CAN HINT:** The 7 rights to medication administration: **R**ight route, **R**ight client, **R**ight drug, **R**ight rationale, **R**ight dose, **R**ight time, and **R**ight documentation

7.19 ③ Option #3 is the correct answer. While all of these need to be administered, the headache is the priority.

7.20 ④ Option #4 is the correct answer. Most cholesterol lowering medications should be taken at night when the liver is "packaging" liver to send out to the blood stream. Options #1, #2, and #3 are incorrect for this medication.

7.21 ② Option #2 is correct. Side effects of Beta 2 agonists include tachycardia and palpitations from the increase SNS stimulus.

7.22 ③ Option #3 is correct since this is on the ISMP publication for dangerous abbreviations. This needs to be spelled out. Options #1, #2, and #4 are incorrect since the drug IU is not spelled out.

7.23 ① Option #1 is correct. The pT should be 1.5–2. 5 times the control. This time is way too long. Options #2, #3, and #4 are all appropriate and do not require questioning.

7.24 ③ Option #3 is the correct answer. Iron causes the stool to turn a greenish black and can give the appearance of blood in the stool. Clients need to know that this may occur. Option #1 is incorrect because it will alter the absorption of the iron. Vitamin C, on the other hand, will enhance the absorption of the iron. Option #2 is incorrect because it does not need to be taken at night. Option #4 is incorrect because enteric coated tablets should not be crushed.

7.25 ① Option #1 is the correct answer. Therapeutic effect is seen when the hematocrit level is between 36 and 52%. Epogen is given for the reversal of anemia associated with clients that have chronic renal failure. Option # 2—Hemoglobin 11–18g/dL is normal. Option #3—Neupogen would be given to increase the WBC not Epogen. WBC level is within normal range of 5,000 to 10,000/mm³. Option #4—Platelet count is within the normal range of 150,000–400,000 cells/mm³.

7.26 ④ Option #4 is the correct answer. Colace is a stool softener that is used to treat constipation. Some of the undesirable effects include abdominal cramps, diarrhea or nausea / vomiting. Option #1—Orange urine is incorrect. Option #2 is not related to this topic. They could have urinary retention or an accumulation of gas in the GI tract. If taking opioid medications, client could have urinary retention. Option #3—HR of 72 is within the normal range of 60 to 80 beats per minute.

7.27 ③ Option #3 is the correct answer. COPD is one of the indications to receive the pneumococcal vaccine before the age of 65 per CDC guidelines. Anyone with cardiopulmonary disease is indicated to receive the pneumococcal vaccine according to JCAHO. Option #1 is incorrect; it only covers 23 purified polysaccharide antigens of S. pneumoniae. Option #2 is incorrect; it is not indicated for children in day care centers. Option #4 is incorrect. "For any person who has received a dose of pneumococcal vaccine at age > 65 years, revaccination is not indicated," per CDC.

7.28 ① Option #1 is correct. Eggs are utilized in the process of manufacturing this vaccine. Options #2, #3, and #4 are incorrect. The influenza vaccine should be given, when indicated, to individuals from September through March. Fatigue and muscle aches are a possible side effect of this vaccine. The influenza vaccine is indicated for clients with HIV and AIDS.

7.29 The correct dosage is 18 units for the regular morning dose plus 12 units for the sliding scale giving a total of 30 units in the syringe.

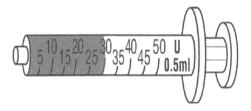

7.30 ② Option #2 is the correct answer. Levothyroxine (Synthroid) raises metabolism which leads to an increase pulse, not a decrease in blood pressure or weight gain. The adverse effect would be an increase in blood pressure and weight loss. The urine output is above the minimum level of 30 mLs per hour.

7.31 ③ Option #3 is the correct answer. Glipizide (Glucotrol) will have an onset within 30 to 60 minutes. If food is not eaten within 30 minutes of taking the medication, the client will experience hypoglycemia. Eating six small meals will maintain a more even blood glucose level versus eating three large meals, but food must still be eaten within 30 minutes of taking the medication no matter how many meals are eaten. Hard candy can be used to raise the blood glucose level when it is low. To alert medical personnel of the presence of diabetes mellitus, the client should purchase the medical identification jewelry and wear.

7.32　①　Option #1 is the correct answer. Prednisone causes the client to retain fluid thus raising the blood pressure and pulse and causing pulmonary edema that can be noted by checking breath sounds for crackles and rales. Option #2 is incorrect because an assessment needs to be made first. Option #3 is not the first action. Option #4 is not the first action.

7.33　④　Option #4 is the correct answer. All of these are problems that can be anticipated as adverse effects including stomach bleeding.

7.34　②　Option #2 is the correct answer. Psyllium is a powder that is taken after being mixed in liquid; if allowed to sit will become solidified.

7.35　③　Option #3 is the correct answer. Diamox is a proximal tubule diuretic. Elderly clients are especially susceptible to hypotension, and hypokalemia while taking this class of drug. Option #1 is incorrect. Increased incontinence is possible with the frail elderly. Offer assistance to the bathroom frequently. Option #2 is incorrect. Diamox must be discontinued gradually to prevent fluid retention. Option #4 is incorrect. Always start at the lowest possible dose for the elderly, and titrate up if needed.

CHAPTER 8

Physiological Integrity
Reduction of Risk Potential

The greatest risk in life is to wait for and depend upon others for your own security.
—Denis Waitley

✔ Clarification of this test ...

The minimum standards include providing appropriate follow-up after incident, urinary catheters, collecting specimens, monitoring lab test/diagnostic results, prenatal complications, client care undergoing treatment, procedures, surgery to reduce complications. Examples of these activities include:

- ☛ Check and monitor client vital signs
- ☛ Perform an electrocardiogram (EKG/ECG)
- ☛ Perform venipuncture for blood draws
- ☛ Perform blood glucose monitoring
- ☛ Maintain central venous catheter
- ☛ Collect specimen for diagnostic testing (i.e., blood, urine, stool, or sputum)
- ☛ Monitor diagnostic and laboratory test results
- ☛ Identify signs and symptoms of potential prenatal complication
- ☛ Perform neurological checks
- ☛ Perform circulatory checks
- ☛ Check for urinary retention (i.e., bladder scan/ultrasound or palpation)
- ☛ Administer and check proper use of compression stockings/sequential compression devices (SCD)
- ☛ Perform risk monitoring and implement interventions
- ☛ Monitor continuous or intermittent suction of nasogastric (NG) tube
- ☛ Implement measures to prevent complication of client condition or procedure (i.e., circulatory complication, seizure, aspiration, or potential neurological disorder)
- ☛ Evaluate client oxygen (O_2) saturation
- ☛ Provide care for client before surgical procedure, including reinforcing teaching
- ☛ Insert, maintain, and remove urinary catheter
- ☛ Insert, maintain, and remove nasogastric (NG) tube
- ☛ Maintain and remove peripheral intravenous (IV) catheter
- ☛ Assist with the performance of a diagnostic or invasive procedure (i.e., call a time-out, bronchoscopy, needle biopsy)

8.1 What plan of care is the priority for a client who is presenting with nausea, diarrhea, muscle weakness, and an abnormal ECG and is taking spironolactone (Aldactone), lisinopril (Zestril), and glipizide (Glucotrol)?

① Report a serum potassium level of 5.2 mEq/L.
② Report a serum sodium level 146 mEq/L.
③ Instruct client about the importance of eating bananas.
④ Assess characteristics of the lips and mucous membranes.

8.2 Which of these nursing actions by the UAP indicates an understanding of the standard of care when preparing a client for a thoracentesis with left-sided empyema?

① Position client in the high-Fowler's position with the lower torso flat.
② Position client in the supine position with the feet elevated.
③ Position client sitting with upper torso over bedside table.
④ Position client on the right side with left knee bent.

8.3 Which of these laboratory reports would be the highest priority to report to the healthcare provider for a client with Addison's disease?

① Blood Urea Nitrogen–6 mg/mL
② Serum potassium–3.1 Eq/L
③ Serum glucose–50 mg/dL
④ Serum sodium–148 mEq/L

8.4 Which statement by the client best indicates an understanding of the preparation for a scheduled magnetic resonance imaging (MRI)?

① "The dye used in the test will turn my urine orange for about 24 hours."
② "I will be put to sleep for this procedure. I will return to my room in 2 to 3 hours."
③ "This procedure will take about 1½ hours to complete. It will be noisy."
④ "The wires that will be attached to my head and chest will not cause me any pain."

8.5 Which of these clinical findings should be reported to the healthcare provider immediately for a client who is being managed and treated for acute low-back pain?

① Discomfort that has lasted approximately 3½ weeks.
② When the leg is elevated, there is pain in the lower back.
③ L4 to L5 has diffuse, aching sensation.
④ A new onset of urinary incontinence.

8.6 Which nursing action indicates the LPN understands how to safely check the placement of the nasogastric tube after it has been inserted?

① Test the pH of the stomach contents and expect the pH to be 5 or greater.
② Inject air into the tube and listen over the lower lung fields.
③ Always do an x-ray confirmation prior to any care with the nasogastric tube.
④ Aspirate gently to collect gastric content and assess color and test pH.

8.7 Which of these nursing actions would be most appropriate when collecting a 24-hour urine specimen diagnostic test?

① Collect all urine voided into a specimen cup.
② Keep all urine collected for 24 hours in a sterile container in the refrigerator.
③ Request client void first into the bedpan and then stop midstream, and finish the voiding into the specimen container.
④ Review the importance of discarding the first voided specimen prior beginning the collection process.

8.8　Which of the nursing actions would be appropriate for the LPN to initiate when placing a catheter in a female client. *Select all that apply.*

① Darken the room.
② Position female client in the semi-Fowler's position with knees bent.
③ Apply sterile drape exposing the urinary meatus.
④ Insert the catheter into the meatus using the sterile hand.
⑤ Maintain surgical aseptic technique during the procedure.

8.9　The LPN is newly employed on the night shift at a long term care facility, and is the only licensed person on this shift. A client was admitted in stable condition after being discharged from the hospital with the diagnosis of COPD exacerbation, NIDDM, depression, chronic renal failure and hypertension. The physician has ordered vital signs every 6 hours. When the nurse enters the client's room at midnight, the client is asleep. What action should the LPN take?

① Obtain vital signs on the client as quickly as possible.
② Delay obtaining vital signs until the client is awake.
③ Delegate the vital signs to a nursing assistant.
④ Document the reason the vital signs were not obtained.

8.10　The LPN is preparing to care for the following client. A 78-year-old man, history of COPD, GERD, HTN, being admitted with severe nausea, vomiting and diarrhea secondary to food poisoning. Vital signs are: BP–102/60, P–88, R–22, and T–99.6°F. Sodium level is 135 mEq/L, potassium 3.1 mEq/L, chloride 104 mEq/L. What equipment is essential for the nurse to have available for this client?

① A telemetry monitor
② Blood pressure cuff
③ Thermometer
④ Bed side commode

8.11　The LPN is working in a busy obstetrician's office. The provider of care has ordered a urine sample to rule out an infection. How should the LPN proceed to obtain the urine sample from the client?

① Clarify the order with the client.
② Use clean technique when obtaining specimen.
③ Collect urine for 24 hours for this specimen.
④ Instruct client to void a bit of urine into commode and then rest of void is caught in a sterile cup.

8.12　The LPN is working on a surgical unit and is caring for a client who is two days postoperative and recovering from a total hip arthroplasty. The client reports to the nurse, "I am having a lot of pain in my lower leg that is different from the pain I have been having. It feels like something is wrong." What immediate action should the LPN take?

① Notify the charge nurse immediately.
② Assess when the client last received pain medication.
③ Evaluate color, motion, pulses in both lower legs of the client.
④ Massage the lower leg to promote client comfort.

8.13　The LPN is assisting with a blood pressure screening clinic. A woman approaches the desk and states, "I would like to have my blood pressure checked, but I have had a bilateral mastectomy. Can my blood pressure still be checked?" How should the LPN respond?

① "Yes, I can check your blood pressure on your arm."
② "Yes, I can check your blood pressure on your wrist."
③ "Yes. I will contact your physician first to check which arm we can use."
④ "Yes, but I will need to check your blood pressure on your leg."

8.14 What client should be assessed initially after report?

① A 1-year-old admitted with otitis media during the last shift.
② A 12-year-old admitted with pneumonia yesterday.
③ A 14-year-old recovering from a fractured femur.
④ A 15-year-old admitted with asthma 45 min. ago and had an exacerbation 15 minutes ago which was relieved by an albuterol inhaler treatment.

8.15 Which of these assessment findings should the LPN report for a client with the diagnosis of pheochromocytoma?

① Blood pressure–98/60 and hot and dry skin.
② Lethargy and complaints of being cold.
③ Blood pressure–160/98 and cardiac palpitations.
④ Headache with a blood pressure of 100/68.

8.16 What would be the priority of care for a client who has a sensory alteration of visual impairment?

① Use flashing lights instead of a warning sound from alarms.
② Remove throw rugs to prevent tripping and falling.
③ Protect and inspect body parts that lack sensation.
④ Make sure smoke detectors are functioning to detect odors that are not perceived.

8.17 A client received 2 extra doses of albuterol for relief of bronchoconstriction from COPD. What would be priority of care?

① Notify provider of care.
② Document bradycardia.
③ Complete appropriate report and document complications of lethargy.
④ Document tachycardia and tremors on incident report and notify provider of care.

8.18 Which nursing action would be most appropriate for the LPN who is performing a fecal occult blood testing (Guaiac test)?

① Instruct client to collect specimen from the toilet.
② With a gloved hand place small amounts of stool on one slide for the diagnostic test.
③ Place a couple of drops of developer on the opposite side of the slide, and if blue color appears, the test is positive for blood.
④ Place stool specimen in a container to take to lab.

8.19 What plan would be most appropriate for collecting a sputum sample for a diagnostic test? Collect the specimen:

① Immediately after respiratory therapy.
② In the evening.
③ First thing in the morning.
④ At noon.

8.20 Which nursing action indicates the LPN understands how to safely position the client for insertion of a nasogastric tube? The LPN positions client in the:

① Fowler's position.
② Semi-Fowler's position.
③ Supine position.
④ Sim's position.

8.21 Which nursing action indicates the LPN understands how to safely use restraints on an elderly client who continues to remove oxygen mask?

① Tie the restraint to side rails.
② Loosen or remove the restraint and test capillary refill, temperature, and pulse every 1–2 hours.
③ Advise provider of care of the need to have an order for the restraints weekly.
④ Restrain with the ability to fit 1 finger between the device and client to prevent injury.

8.22 The provider of care has ordered a Nonstress testing be performed on a woman who is 36 weeks pregnant. The LPN is preparing the client for the procedure. Which statement made by the client evaluates the client's understanding of the procedure?

① "I need to remain NPO for 6 hours after the procedure."
② "I will need to lie on my back for 1 hour after the procedure."
③ "There is no special preparation for the test."
④ "I will need someone to drive me home afterwards."

8.23 The LPN is reinforcing teaching to a pregnant woman. Which statement made by the client would alert the nurse that additional information was needed?

① "I should report a fever immediately."
② "A slight headache is not of concern."
③ "I will call if I develop swelling of my hands or face."
④ "I should not have any visual changes."

8.24 The client is admitted to the emergency department with confusion and is unable to remember their last name, date, or the name of the city. The client's spouse reports that the client was "fine yesterday". What finding made could explain the reason for the acute confusion?

① Family history of Alzheimer's disease
② History of hypertension
③ Oxygen saturation of 94%
④ Sodium level of 131 mEq / L

8.25 The LPN receives a call from the laboratory personnel with an abnormal lab value. Which of the following reports would be of greatest concern to the LPN?

① A client with diabetes who has a blood sugar of 212 mg/dL.
② An end stage renal client with a potassium level of 5.9 mEq/L.
③ A client with a cardiac dysrhythmia who has a sodium level of 139 mEq/L.
④ A post-partum mother with a hematocrit of 41%.

8.26 What would be the priority of care for a client during a seizure?

① Complete and thorough documentation.
② Check all equipment to make certain it is functioning appropriately.
③ Protect head, provide privacy and loosen clothing.
④ Explain to family what happened during the seizure.

8.27 What nursing action should be the priority for a client with a spinal cord injury at T_6 who complains about a throbbing headache that just started? The clinical assessment reveals BP–180/94, HR–48 BPM, diaphoresis, and flushing of the neck and face.

① Reposition client carefully upright and lower legs if possible.
② Assess for sensory loss.
③ Administer morphine for complaints of headache.
④ Notify the HCP regarding the change in clinical status.

8.28 The LPN is working on a medical surgical unit and a client has returned following a bowel resection. As the LPN makes AM rounds, the client is observed becoming restless. What nursing action would be the priority for the LPN to implement?

① Administer pain medication as ordered.
② Assess vital signs and urine output.
③ Ask family if client has a history of drug or alcohol abuse.
④ Order stat labs for electrolytes and blood gases.

8.29 For a client with a neurological disorder, which nursing assessment would be most helpful in determining subtle changes in the client's level of consciousness?

① Client posturing
② Glasgow Coma Scale
③ Client thinking pattern
④ Occurrence of hallucinations

8.30 Which of these 80-year-old clients should be referred to the provider of care for further evaluation?

① A client with presbyopia.
② A client with presbycusis.
③ A client with a decreased sensitivity in cranial nerve 1.
④ A client with a depressed cranial nerve 9 and 10.

8.31 Which of these clients would be the priority to be assessed immediately following report?

① A client with a brain tumor who is complaining of a headache, with BP–170/58 mm Hg, HR–50 BPM, and motor, verbal and eye opening responses to deep pain only.
② A client with a spinal cord injury who has a BP–138, HR–80, Glasgow Coma Scale–12.
③ A client who is 1 hour post-seizure and is resting on side with SaO_2 95%, but is lethargic.
④ A client with a spinal cord injury at T_6 with altered sensation in lower extremities.

8.32 The LPN is caring for a client who has been immobilized for 3 days following a perineal prostatectomy. The client begins to experience sudden shortness of breath, chest pain, and coughing with blood-tinged sputum. Immediate nursing actions would include:

① Assist the client to cough. If unsuccessful, then suction.
② Elevate the head of the bed, begin oxygen, and further assess respiratory status.
③ Position in supine position with legs elevated. Monitor CVP closely.
④ Administer morphine for chest pain. Obtain a 12 lead ECG to evaluate cardiac status.

8.33 Which of these nursing actions represent an understanding of how to successfully set up a sterile field?

① Place all supplies as close to edge as possible.
② Wear gown and gloves at all times.
③ Set up the field above waist level.
④ Open supplies with sterile gloves.

8.34 The pulse oximeter alarms indicating the oxygen saturation is at 86%. What would be the priority action?

① Administering oxygen via mask.
② Checking the position of the probe.
③ Resetting the pulse oximeter's alarm.
④ Completing a cardiovascular assessment.

8.35 Which of these consistent observations would be most important for the nurse to document and report to the charge nurse?

① The UAP assists the client to wash paste out of hair following an EEG.
② The UAP assists the male client following a cardiac catheterization to use the urinal.
③ The UAP assists the RN to place client in the side lying position following a seizure
④ The UAP assists the client to the bathroom following a lumbar puncture.

ANSWERS & RATIONALES

8.1 ① The correct answer is Option #1. Aldactone is a potassium-sparing diuretic, and when given with Zestril, there is a potential problem with hyperkalemia. Option #1 is the answer due to the potassium level. (normal: 3.5–5.0 mEq/L). Option #2 is not the priority over option #1. In fact with the clinical presentation, the sodium would be low. (normal: 135–145 mEq/L). Option #3 is incorrect since these foods are high in potassium and could result in hyperkalemia. While Option #4 is appropriate, it is not a priority to option #1.

 I CAN HINT: Ace inhibitors, such as lisinopril (Zestril), inhibit angiotensin-converting enzyme (ACE), preventing conversion of angiotensin I to angiotensin II (reduced formation of angiotensin II decreases peripheral arterial resistance, thus decreasing aldosterone secretion). Spironolactone (Aldactone) promotes excretion of sodium and water, but retains potassium in the distal renal tubule. An easy way to remember Aldactone is think of "Alan at the commode holding on to a piggy bank which is a "postassium bank" and think of him taking a "LEAK".

Low Na⁺

Elevated T waves from ↑ K⁺

Agranulocytosis with triamterene

K⁺ must be monitored for hyperkalemia

8.2 ③ Option #3 is correct for this procedure with a left-sided empyema for a thoracentesis. This position over the bedside table allows the ribs to separate, which assists the provider of care in positioning the needle into the pleural cavity. If the client is unable to assume this position, then the client is placed on the affected side with the head of bed slightly elevated. The purpose for this alternate position is that the fluid will be dependent. Options #1, #2, and #4 are incorrect for this procedure.

 I CAN HINT: The NCLEX® Activity that this question is testing is "Position client to prevent complications with tests, treatments, or procedures." "ACT NOW" will assist you in organizing additional information for these pretest preparations for the diagnostic procedures.

Allergies

Consent

Teaching

NPO

p**O**sition

Watch vital signs; symptoms of complications

 I CAN HINT: Another strategy to assist you on the NCLEX® with answering these questions regarding thoracentesis is to remember this diagnostic test is implemented by aspirating fluid from the pleural cavity. This can be used for both diagnostic and therapeutic purposes. "**CENTESIS**" will assist you in organizing the key concepts for this procedure.

Consent after client understands the procedure

Explain procedure to client

Note, ideally client would be positioned on the side of the bed with the arms and head over the bedside table.

The vital signs should be assessed for any trends prior to, during, and after procedure (bleeding, breathing)

Elevate HOB slightly and place on affected side if client is unable to assume sitting position

So, the area containing the fluid that will be aspirated should be dependent

Infuse cytotoxic drugs into the pleural space if client has a malignancy

Side up with puncture side (or in semi-Fowler's position) and monitor respiratory status, breath sounds for possible pneumothorax, and / or bleeding; Support and reassure client during procedure

8.3 ③ Option #3 is correct. Decreased hepatic gluconeogenesis and increased tissue glucose uptake may result in hypoglycemia in clients with Addison's disease. Option #1 is incorrect. There may actually be an elevation in the BUN and other waste products, since there may be a decreased renal perfusion. Option #2 is incorrect. Serum potassium actually may be increased with Addison's disease, and option #4 is incorrect, since the sodium is typically decreased.

 I CAN HINT: Addison's disease is caused by a decrease in secretion of the adrenal cortex hormones. There is a decrease physiologic response to stress, vascular insufficiency, and hypoglycemia. There is a decrease in the aldosterone secretions (mineral corticoids), which normally promote concentration of sodium and water and excretion of potassium. As a result of this, the sodium may be low and potassium elevated. Now that you understand the pathophysiology that is occurring with Addison's disease; let us provide you with a great memory strategy.

Remember the saying, "**Some People Get Cold**". Think of the "S" as Sodium, "P" as Potassium, "G" as Glucose, and "C" as Calcium. Now, remember there is a "**D**" in **Add**ison's disease, so we will start with the arrows going **DOWN** and then every other direction. Here you go!

Sodium ↓

Potassium ↑

Glucose ↓

Calcium ↑

See how EASY this is!!!! We hope you will NEVER forget this. This is what we call moving information to the long-term memory!

8.4 ③ Option #3 is correct. This diagnostic test will take approximately 1 hour and it is noisy, so earplugs or sedation may be provided. The client must lie supine with the head stabilized. Client should remove all jewelry prior to the procedure. A hospital gown is worn to prevent any metals from interfering with the magnet. If sedation is expected, the client should be NPO for 4 to 8 hours prior to the procedure. Determine if the client has a history of claustrophobia and explain the tight space and noise. All jewelry, pagers, and phones should be removed by healthcare provider and family members who are in the scanning area while the magnet is on. Since the procedure is performed with the client in a supine position, the nurse may place pillows in the small of the client's back that may assist in preventing back pain. The head must be secured to prevent unnecessary movement during the procedure. Option #1 is incorrect. Option #2 is incorrect since the client is not put to sleep. The client may receive some sedation, but the client will not be in procedure for 2-3 hours. Option #4 is incorrect for this procedure.

 I CAN HINT: "ACT NOW" will assist you in organizing the concepts for diagnostic procedures.

Assess understanding of procedure

Consent

Teach about the time for completing the procedure and the noise involved

NPO

p**O**sition during and/or following the procedure

Watch for complications such as from bleeding, anxiety, breathing, etc.

8.5 ④ Option #4 is correct. This is a neurologic change and symptoms such as bladder or bowel changes or foot-drop should be reported to the healthcare provider immediately. Option #1 is incorrect, since when a client experiences acute low back pain, these symptoms may take 4 to 6 weeks to resolve. Options #2 and #3 are not findings that should be reported immediately. The client may present with both of these symptoms when there is a problem with acute low back pain.

 I CAN HINT: The key to success with this question, as with many of the NCLEX® questions, it to remember that an "expected outcome" is most likely not going to be the priority to report or intervene with immediately! Options #2 and #3 are expected findings with acute low back pain.

8.6 ④ The correct answer is Option #4. The pH should be 4 or less. Option #1 is incorrect because the pH should be 4 or less. Options #2 and #3 are inappropriate practice.

8.7 ④ Option #4 is the correct answer. The first voiding of the 24-hour urine specimen is discarded and then the test begins at this time. All the specimens are kept after this on ice. If there is an order for a urinalysis, the client will collect urine in a specimen container. If a culture is ordered, client will void first into the toilet, and then stop midstream and collect remaining specimen in the container.

8.8 ③ Options #3, #4, and #5 are correct
④ nursing actions for this procedure to
⑤ decrease the risk of infection. Option #1 is not appropriate. In fact, it is important to establish a good light source to visualize the perineal area. Option #2 is inappropriate. The client should be positioned in the supine position with the knees bent and apart to facilitate insertion of the catheter.

8.9 ① Option #1 is the correct answer. The physician has an order, and this is a newly admitted client from the hospital. It is imperative that the LPN assess the vital signs. If the nurse initiates this order in a timely manner, there will be less interruption in client's sleep pattern. Options #2, #3, and #4 delay the order to obtain the vital signs, which is not prudent nursing care.

8.10 ① Option #1 is the correct answer. In the client assessment information, the client has decreased potassium which can cause a life threatening arrhythmia. (Normal serum potassium, 3.5 – 5.0 mEq / L) All other lab values are within normal range. Options #2, #3, and #4 are equipment that will be needed for care of the client; however, the most essential equipment to have for this client is a continuous ECG monitor to monitor for an arrhythmia as a result of the hypokalemia. (Refer to *Nursing Made Insanely Easy*, Rayfield & Manning for the memory strategy of the **Magic 4's** that will help you EASILY remember your lab values!)

8.11 ④ Option #4 is the correct answer. This technique is appropriate for a specimen evaluating a culture and sensitivity which is what must be done for a client with an infection. Options #1, #2, and #3 are incorrect for this client. If there is a need for order clarification, this should be done with the provider of care.

8.12 ③ Option #3 is the correct answer, as this allows the nurse to determine if the new complaint is related to a circulatory impairment, or part of the surgical recovery. Option #1 is incorrect, as the LPN must assess the client complaints to determine what is needed. Option #2 is incorrect, as any complaint of pain must be assessed prior to administering pain medication. Option #4 is incorrect. The nurse must assess the lower leg and determine if the client could have a circulatory impairment, and until that assessment is made, massaging is contraindicated. This nursing action could result in dislodging a clot.

8.13 ④ Option #4 is the correct answer. Option #1 is inappropriate, as the nurse should not perform blood pressures on the arm of a mastectomy client. Option #2 is incorrect. Option #3 is not warranted, as the nurse can evaluate blood pressure, however, the safest method to do this is by checking blood pressure on the client's leg.

8.14 ④ Option #4 is the correct answer. This client experienced a major airway complication that required a pharmacological intervention. The nurse needs to evaluate client for desired outcomes from the medication as well as potential adverse effects from the albuterol. Option #1 is not correct. While otitis media is a concern for this client, it is not a priority over an airway issue. Option #2 is a concern, but there is no assessment to mandate this client to be a priority over option #4. Option #3 is recovering from the fracture and has no assessment findings indicating any complication.

8.15 ③ Option #3 is the correct answer. Clients with pheochromocytoma produce and store catecholamines, such as epinephrine and norepinephrine. The excess epinephrine and norepinephrine produce sympathetic nervous system effects. Hypertensive crisis is the most significant complication of a pheochromocytoma. The nurse must monitor the client's blood pressure and observe for any signs or symptoms that may indicate a hypertensive crisis. Other signs and symptoms of this disorder may include: pain in chest / abdomen accompanied by nausea and vomiting, headache, palpitations, diaphoresis, heat intolerance, tremors, apprehension. Option #1 is incorrect because the concern is not with a low but a high blood pressure and the skin does not get hot and dry, but diaphoretic. Option #2 is incorrect. The client would experience heat intolerance and apprehension. Option #4 is not totally correct. The headache is correct, but the blood pressure in not a concern.

8.16 ② Option #2 is correct for clients who are visually impaired. Option #1 would be appropriate for clients who experience an auditory impairment. Option #3 would be appropriate for a client with a tactile impairment (paresthesia). Option #4 would be appropriate for a client with an impairment of the olfactory senses.

8.17 ④ Option #4 is correct. An overdose of a Beta 2 Adrenergic Agonist may result in tachycardia, hypertension, tremors, and / or cardiac dysrhythmias. Option #1 is incorrect since there is no assessment to share with the provider of care. Option #2 is incorrect for this medication; it would be tachycardia versus bradycardia. The documentation must reflect the appropriate complication for this drug classification. Option #3 is also incorrect as is #2.

8.18 ③ Option #3 is a correct nursing action. Option #1 is incorrect. If able, ask client to collect specimen in the toilet receptacle, bedpan, or bedside commode. Option #2 is incorrect. The specimen should be applied with a wooden applicator versus the gloved hand. Option #4 would be appropriate for a stool for culture, parasites, and ova versus for a Guaiac test.

8.19 ③ Option #3 is correct. This is the time of the day for the collecting the best specimen. Options #1, #2, and #4 are incorrect.

8.20 ① Option #1 is correct. This position facilitates the tube going in. Other options are incorrect.

8.21 ② Option #2 is correct. It is imperative to assess for any neurological or circulatory deficits routinely based on hospital protocol. Option #1 is unsafe. Restraints should be loosely knotted, so they can be easily removed and tied to the bed frame, not on the rails, which can hurt client when the rails are lowered. Option #3 is incorrect. The order needs to be done every 24 hours. Option #4 is incorrect. Two fingers should be able to go between the device and client to prevent injury.

8.22 ③ Option #3 is correct. A Nonstress test requires a woman to sit in a recliner or bed, in the semi-Fowler's position for 30 minutes, while an external monitor is placed on the client to evaluate the fetal heart rate in response to activity. Option #2 is incorrect (pregnant women should not lie on their back). Option #4 is incorrect, as the client is not receiving sedation.

8.23 ② Option #2 is the correct answer. Option #2 (headache) may indicate an elevated blood pressure. If the pregnant woman believes a headache is ok, then she needs additional teaching! Pain is subjective, and what is slight for one pregnant woman may be severe for a different pregnant woman. If the mother believes this is acceptable, this is a priority concern due to the risks that may be involved with this clinical finding in a pregnant client. Option #1 is appropriate, as it is not normal to have a fever, and is of concern in the pregnant woman. Option #3 is appropriate. This needs to be reported. Swelling of the hands and face may be a symptom of pre-eclampsia. Option #4 is a correct statement as well. Visual changes may indicate an elevated blood pressure.

8.24 ④ Option #4 is the correct answer. A low sodium level, as indicated by option #4, can result in acute confusion and is the most clinically significant finding. Alzheimer's disease does not cause acute confusion and takes time to develop. The fact the spouse reports the client was "fine yesterday" indicates an acute process. Option #2 is incorrect. Option #3 is a low level, and may be indicative of a disease process, but is not as significant as Option #4.

8.25 ② Option #2 is the correct answer. Option #2 represents an elevated potassium level which can result in life threatening cardiac dysrhythmias. Option #1 does present an elevated blood glucose level, however, a level of 212 mg /dL is not a priority over option #2. Option #3 represents a normal sodium level. Option #4 represents a normal hematocrit.

8.26 ③ Option #3 is correct for a client during a seizure. Safety is a priority! Option #1 should occur following the seizure. Option #2 should occur when client is admitted with this diagnosis and prior to the seizure. A major responsibility of the nurse is to assure that ALL equipment is working appropriately prior to needing to use it! Option #4 would occur following the seizure versus during the seizure.

8.27 ① Option #1 is the correct answer. This client is presenting with autonomic dysreflexia. This medical condition may occur with spinal cord injuries at T_6 or higher. The typical causes include a full bladder, fecal impaction, or a funning feeling with the skin. The assessment findings are reflected in this question. It is important to reposition the client upright as outlined in option #1 with careful attention to not manipulate and change alignment of the spinal cord. The care then includes removing the cause and administering an antihypertensive medication. (Refer to *Nursing Made Insanely Easy*, by Rayfield & Manning, for the memory strategy to assist in EASILY remembering this concept.) Option #2 is incorrect. Option #3 is contraindicated for these clients. Option #4 in not a priority over option #1. The situation requires immediate intervention

with the client due to the crisis. The follow through with the healthcare provider will be implemented, but not first.

8.28 ② Option #2 is correct. Post-operative restlessness should create a high degree of suspicion of hypoxemia (i.e., due to bleeding). Vital signs and urine output will give information regarding intravascular volume. Option #1 requires further assessment to rule out hypoxemia as the cause of the restlessness. Option #3 may indicate an erroneous assumption. Option #4 might be the second priority, but is not a priority to option #2.

8.29 ② Option #2 is correct. The Glasgow Coma Scale score best evaluates changes in a client's level of consciousness by evaluating eye opening, motor, and verbal response. Option #1 indicates increased intracranial pressure. Options #3 and #4 are more appropriate for the psychiatric client.

8.30 ④ Option #4 is correct because it is a concern due to the risk with gagging. The glossopharyngeal (swallowing / gag reflex) and the vagus nerves assist with swallowing. Options #1, #2, and #3 are normal changes with the aging process.

8.31 ① Option #1 is correct. This client is exhibiting signs of increased intracranial pressure and mandates immediate care. Option #2 is stable and is not a priority over option #1. Option #3 is an expected finding following a seizure and is not a priority over #1. Option #4 is an expected finding with this level of spinal injury, and does not require immediate attention.

8.32 ② Option #2 is correct answer. Based on the client's history, current immobility, and assessment factors, this client may be experiencing a pulmonary emboli. Priority nursing care is to prevent severe hypoxia and maintain ventilation. Option #1 is inappropriate and does not address the client's current clinical findings. Option #3 is for hypotension and would not be appropriate for this client. Option #4 is for a cardiac client who may be presenting with signs of a myocardial infarction.

8.33 ③ Option #3 is correct. Sterile fields should be set up above the waist. Option #1 will not maintain sterility. Option #2 is incorrect because gowns are not always necessary. Option #4 is incorrect because the supplies can be opened with bare hands, but touched inside the package with sterile gloves.

8.34 ② Option #2 is correct. The probe may have fallen off. This is the priority action to prevent inappropriate or unnecessary intervention. Options #1, #3, and #4 are incorrect.

8.35 ④ Option #4 is correct. This action represents unsafe practice since the client following a lumbar puncture should remain in the bed for a designated period of time. Options # 1, #2, and #3 represent safe nursing practice, and do not require the nurse to document and report to the charge nurse.

CHAPTER 9

Physiological Integrity
Physiological Adaptation

The measure of intelligence is the ability to change.
—Albert Einstein

✔ Clarification of this test ...

The minimum standards include providing direct care for clients with acute, chronic, or life-threatening conditions, ostomy care, ventilator care, illness management and emergencies. Examples of these activities include:

- Identify/intervene to control signs of hypoglycemia or hyperglycemia
- Recognize and report basic abnormalities on a client cardiac monitor strip
- Provide care for client drainage device (i.e., wound drain or chest tube)
- Provide cooling/warming measures to restore normal temperature
- Provide care for a client with a tracheostomy
- Provide care for a client with an ostomy (i.e., colostomy, ileostomy, or urostomy)
- Provide care for a client on a ventilator
- Perform wound care and/or dressing change
- Perform check of client pacemaker
- Perform care for client after surgical procedure
- Remove wound sutures or staples
- Remove client wound drainage device
- Intervene to improve client respiratory status (i.e., breathing treatment, suctioning or repositioning)
- Reinforce education to client regarding care and condition
- Identify signs and symptoms related to an acute or chronic illness
- Respond/intervene to a client life-threatening situation (i.e., cardiopulmonary resuscitation)
- Recognize and report change in client condition

9.1 What is the priority for the postoperative nursing care for a client who has a new ileostomy?

① Irrigate the ileostomy consistently every A.M.
② Change the ostomy bag when it is about one-third full.
③ Irrigate with 500 to 1000 mL of warm tap water.
④ Change the appliance every 8 hours to prevent contamination.

9.2 A client with a permanent colostomy on the transverse colon questions the nurse as to whether or not he will ever be able to establish bowel control. The nursing response would be based on which concept?

① There is little chance that the client will gain an adequate control with this colostomy.
② Control may be achieved with colostomy irrigations twice a day.
③ Daily colostomy irrigations and diet are frequently used to maintain colostomy control.
④ A high residue diet that provides bulk to the stool may be used to maintain bowel control.

9.3 At the time of diagnosis, a client with Bell's Palsy is given a supply of eye patches. What would be most important to caution client against?

① Allowing the cornea of the eye to become dry.
② Photosensitivity regarding light on the retina.
③ Sudden movement of the head when bending over.
④ Contamination from the affected eye to the other eye.

9.4 A client recovering from Streptococcal pneumonia has a chest x-ray which reveals a higher degree of atelectasis in the right lower lobe. Which nursing intervention would be most appropriate?

① Instruct the client to take deep breaths more frequently.
② Reposition client every hour to the right side.
③ Increase frequency of incentive spirometry.
④ Change respiratory treatment to every 2 hours.

9.5 The LPN should intervene if which of the following actions occur when the unlicensed assistive personnel (UAP) is providing a bed bath to a client who is incontinent?

① The UAP positions client on the right side, with the head of the bed elevated.
② The UAP positions an incontinent diaper under client.
③ The UAP opens the bathroom door when wearing gloves.
④ The UAP log rolls client to provide back care.

9.6 Which of these clinical findings would be a priority for the LPN to report to the provider of care?

① An 80-year-old client presenting with some incontinence when coughing.
② An 82-year-old client with osteoarthritis who complains of stiffness upon awakening in the A.M.
③ An 84-year-old client presenting with a new symptom of incontinence with acute confusion
④ An 86-year-old client, who is taking Digoxin, with a HR–64 BPM.

9.7 Which clinical finding should be reported to the healthcare provider (HCP) following a bronchoscopy?

① Presenting with a depressed gag reflex.
② Coughing up small amounts of blood tinged sputum.
③ Complaining of a sore throat.
④ Presenting with hemoptysis.

9.8 Which of these clients would need nursing intervention immediately after report?

① A 10-year-old client who is post-operative and has received half of a unit of packed red blood cells.

② A 15-year-old client in sickle-cell crisis who has an IV that has infiltrated.

③ A 20-year-old client who needs teaching prior to going for an electroencephalogram (EEG) in the A.M.

④ A 25-year-old client who needs an IV started for surgery in 2 hours.

9.9 One hour in the postoperative period for a client who has a subtotal gastric resection, the client's vital signs are: BP–100/60, HR–88 beats per minute, RR–22, and urine output 40 mL/hour. What should be the initial nursing intervention?

① Maintain a CVP reading of 6–12 mm H_2O pressure.

② Administer nifedipine (Procardia) as ordered.

③ Position client in the Trendelenburg position.

④ Notify physician regarding the urine output.

9.10 What nursing action would the nurse implement next after applying oxygen at 4 liters per nasal cannula for a client who awakens during the night with dyspnea, RR–34, anxiety, jugular vein distension (JVD), and frothy pink sputum?

① Notify physician regarding the change in client's condition.

② Elevate the legs and position 2 pillows behind head of client.

③ Increase IV fluids to liquefy the secretions.

④ Provide privacy by placing client away from the nurses' station.

9.11 Which of these clinical situations should the charge nurse intervene with immediately?

① The LPN is log rolling a client following scoliosis repair.

② The LPN is preparing to administer insulin to a client who is cold and clammy.

③ The LPN is checking the gag reflex prior to giving fluids to client following a bronchoscopy.

④ The LPN is withholding the furosemide (Lasix) for a client complaining of tinnitus and notifying provider of care.

9.12 The nurse has a client with an order to, "Irrigate wound with normal saline, then pack with a damp dressing and cover BID." The nurse plans to perform the dressing change after the morning medications have been passed. What would warrant a change in time plan for the dressing change? The UAP reports:

① AM care has been performed on the client.

② The client has requested a pain medication.

③ The client accidentally spilled the water pitcher and client is soaked.

④ The client is ready for the dressing change.

9.13 While a client is being turned, the client becomes extubated resulting in cyanosis and bradycardia along with some dysrhythmias. What would be the priority nursing action for this client while waiting for the provider of care to arrive?

① Maintain the airway and provide oxygen.

② Begin CPR immediately.

③ Increase the IV fluids.

④ Prepare the medications for resuscitation.

9.14 Which plan would be a priority in an emergency wound evisceration?

① Maintain moisture to the wound.

② Start an IV and begin antibiotics.

③ Keep a sterile dressing over the wound.

④ Irrigate the wound with normal saline.

9.15 Organize the following steps to suctioning in chronological order (with 1 being the first step in this procedure).

① Put on sterile gloves.

② Lubricate catheter with normal saline.

③ Apply suction for 5–10 seconds when removing the catheter.

④ Explain procedure to client.

⑤ Wash hands thoroughly.

9.16 In evaluating the effectiveness of teaching a client with a permanent-demand pacemaker, the client should state that feelings of fainting, dizziness and a slow irregular pulse most likely indicate:

① Failure of the pacemaker battery.
② Competition between the heart and the pacemaker.
③ Occurrence of pericardial tamponade.
④ A rejection of the foreign body.

9.17 A client is one day post-operative after an abdominal hysterectomy and is being evaluated for discharge from the hospital. The LPN identifies edema in the client's right leg. The nurse should:

① Advise client to increase the frequency of post-op leg exercises.
② Consult the client's chart for a history of renal failure or heart failure.
③ Elevate the foot of the client's bed at least thirty degrees.
④ Measure both legs at mid-thigh and mid-calf.

9.18 What action should a nurse take if a pleur-evac attached to a chest tube breaks?

① Immediately clamp the chest tube.
② Notify the physician.
③ Place the end of the tube in sterile water.
④ Reposition the client in the Fowler's position.

9.19 Which finding would the LPN identify as interfering with the effective functioning of chest tubes?

① 15 cm water suction in chest tube system.
② An air leak in water seal chamber.
③ Leaking blood around chest tube site.
④ Clots of blood in the chest tube.

9.20 The nurse assesses a prolonged late deceleration of the fetal heart rate while client is receiving oxytocin (Pitocin) to stimulate labor. The priority nursing intervention would be to:

① Turn off the oxytocin infusion.
② Turn client to left.
③ Change the fluids to Ringer's Lactate.
④ Increase mainline IV rate.

9.21 What assessment should the LPN make for a client who is on a volume cycled positive pressure ventilator and the low pressure alarm sounds?

① Client is biting on the tubing.
② Excessive fluid is in the ventilator tubing.
③ A leak in the client's endotracheal tube cuff.
④ Client is lying on the tubing.

9.22 An elderly client with COPD in the long term facility becomes confused and restless. What would be the priority of care for the LPN to implement with this client?

① Assess the client's sodium and potassium level.
② Evaluate the client's temperature.
③ Increase the oxygen flow rate to 6 L / min.
④ Encourage client to perform pursed-lip breathing.

9.23 During rounds in the long term facility, the LPN observes a client with chronic bronchitis experiencing dyspnea, shortness of breath, and a respiratory rate of 32. What position would indicate the nurse understands how to safety care of this client?

① High-Fowler's
② Side-lying
③ Semi-Fowler's
④ Supine

9.24 The LPN is caring for a man, in the long-term facility, who has a double-lumen tracheostomy tube with a cuff. Which of these nursing interventions indicate an understanding of how to provide safe care to this client?

① Maintain the inner cannula of the tracheostomy in place at all times.
② Change the tracheostomy ties every 48 hours.
③ Change the tracheostomy dressing every 8 hours and PRN.
④ Discontinue humidity to prevent dressing saturation.

9.25 A client presents with chest pain after some strenuous activity in the assisted living center. The pain is relieved with nitroglycerine. Which of these cardiac dysrhythmias would reflect this problem?

① Spiked T wave.
② Depressed T wave.
③ Depressed ST segment.
④ Prolonged PR interval.

9.26 A client with type 1 diabetes (IDDM), in the long term facility, presents with nausea, vomiting, and abdominal pain, poor skin turgor, dry mucous membranes, and fruity breath odor. Which additional clinical findings should the LPN monitor indicating a major potential complication for this client?

① Confusion, anxiety, hunger.
② Temperature and lymphadenopathy.
③ Dehydration, abdominal discomfort, hyperpyrexia.
④ Polyuria, polydipsia, nausea and vomiting, weight loss, and hypotension.

9.27 During the first 24 hours after total parenteral nutrition (TPN) therapy is started, the nurse should:

① Monitor vital signs every 3 hours.
② Determine urinalysis results.
③ Evaluate blood glucose levels.
④ Compare weight with previous weight record.

9.28 Prior to administering an IV antibiotic that is ordered, what would be the priority of care for this client?

① Check the IV site for infiltration.
② Do a complete physical assessment.
③ Check vital signs.
④ Evaluate symptoms of an allergic reaction.

9.29 A client is recovering from post GI surgery with a chest x-ray which reveals a higher degree of atelectasis in the right lower lobe. Which nursing intervention would be the most appropriate?

① Instruct the client to take deep breaths more frequently.
② Reposition client every hour to the right side.
③ Increase frequency of incentive spirometry.
④ Change respiratory treatment to every two hours.

9.30 After surgery, the client becomes restless and confused. What is the priority action?

① Administer a pain medicine.
② Order a stat chest x-ray.
③ Assess for drug abuse.
④ Assess vital signs and urine output.

9.31 What is the priority nursing intervention to be included in the preoperative teaching plan for a client scheduled for a cholecystectomy?

① Assessing the client's understanding of the surgical procedure.
② Educating client regarding fluid restrictions.
③ Reviewing how to do leg exercises.
④ Teaching coughing and deep breathing exercises.

9.32 At 4:30 PM a client presents with confusion and diaphoresis after receiving 9 units of NPH insulin at 8:30 AM. What would be the priority nursing intervention?

① Administer 6 oz. of skim milk.
② Evaluate urine for ketones.
③ Evaluate vital signs.
④ Notify provider of care.

9.33 Which of these clients should be seen first immediately after shift report?

   ① A 25-year-old client admitted with a post-op appendectomy with a 1 cm. in diameter of serosanguinous drainage on the dressing.

   ② A 45-year-old client admitted following a hysterectomy 2 days ago and is complaining of chills.

   ③ A 55-year-old client admitted following a motor vehicle accident with a fractured femur and is in Russell's traction.

   ④ A 65-year-old diagnosed with Parkinson's disease.

9.34 A seventy-year-old client is found by the LPN on the floor next to his bed in a Long Term Health Care Facility. He has a history of COPD and coronary artery disease. He is taking antibiotics for his pneumonia. What would be the priority nursing action?'

   ① Immediately begin chest percussions.

   ② Check the presence or absence of pulses.

   ③ Evaluate for unresponsiveness.

   ④ Help client to stand up.

9.35 A client with a history of HTN, COPD, diabetes, and chronic pancreatitis secondary to alcohol abuse is admitted to the emergency department with probable pneumonia. Which assessment finding made by the LPN is of greatest concern?

   ① Oxygen saturation of 89%.

   ② Fasting blood sugar of 204 mg/dL.

   ③ Increased anxiety and agitation.

   ④ SOB on exertion.

I CAN Publishing®, INC.

ANSWERS & RATIONALES

9.1 ② Option #2 is correct. Ostomy bags should be changed when about one-third full to avoid weight of bag dislodging skin barrier. Option #1 is incorrect because an ileostomy should not be irrigated. Option #3 is incorrect since the ileostomy should not be irrigated. This is the correct amount of fluid to irrigate with, however, for a colostomy. Option #4 is incorrect. The appliance should be changed only when it begins to leak or becomes dislodged.

 I CAN HINT: "STOMA" will help you remember the nursing care for an ileostomy.

Stoma should be evaluated every 8 hours after surgery. Should remain pink and moist. (*Dark blue stoma indicates ischemia.*)

The abdominal incision should not get contaminated. Keep the skin around the stoma clean, dry, and free of stool and intestinal secretions. The ileostomy should NOT be irrigated.

Only change skin appliance when it begins to leak or becomes dislodged. Ostomy bags should be changed when about one-third full to avoid weight of bag dislodging skin barrier.

Mild to moderate swelling is common for the first 2 to 3 weeks after surgery, which necessitates changes in size of the appliance

Appliance should fit easily around the stoma and cover all healthy skin.

9.2 ③ Option #3 is correct. Diet and irrigations are the common methods used for colostomy control. Option #1 is incorrect because clients gradually are able to "control" and adapt to their individual bowel evacuation routines. Option #2 is incorrect because irrigation of the colostomy is usually needed only once a day. Option #4 is incorrect because diet may assist in control, but cannot be used alone, and irrigations are more successful.

 I CAN HINT: This is evaluating the NCLEX® activity of "ostomy care". The seven "**DO NOT'S**" will assist you in your clinical decision making about irritating a colostomy. Do NOT:

- Use an enema tube/catheter.
- Irrigate more than once a day.
- Irrigate in the presence of diarrhea.
- Position in the supine but in a sitting position, preferably in the bathroom with the irrigation sleeve in toilet.
- Elevate the solution container for irrigating above 20 inches. (*Do: Elevate approximately 12 to 20 inches and allow solution to flow in gently.*)
- Keep on irrigating if cramping occurs, but instead lower fluid or clamp the tubing. Do not resume until cramping has passed.
- Send client home without teaching about colostomy irrigation.

9.3 ① Option #1 is correct. Paralysis of the eyelid allows the cornea to dry. Patches can be used to keep the eyelid closed to prevent damage. Drops and/or ointments are also used to reduce the chance of corneal damage. Option #2 is incorrect because the problem, properly managed, should not result in a problem with light. Option #3 is for clients with increased intraocular pressure. Option #4 is incorrect because Bell's Palsy is not contagious.

 I CAN HINT: Bell's Palsy is a transient cranial nerve disorder affecting the facial nerve (cranial nerve VII), characterized by a disruption of the motor branches on one side of the face, which results in muscle weakness or flaccidity on the affected side. Changes in physical appearance may be dramatic. This condition is self-limiting with minimal, if any, residual effects. Client may require counseling, if change in facial appearance is permanent. Due to the physical changes that may occur, we use the mnemonic "**IMAGE**" to assist you in remembering the nursing interventions for Bell's Palsy.

Image is a major concern

Methylcellulose drops frequently during the day

Analgesics to decrease pain; as function returns, active facial exercises may be performed

Give eye care; ophthalmic ointment and eye patches may be required at night

Evaluate ability to eat

9.4 ③ Option #3 is correct. Incentive spirometry is a quantifiable method to assess respiratory effort with deep breathing exercises. Increasing the frequency would be a sound nursing decision in an effort to improve the client's pulmonary status. Option #1 would be effective, however, not as much as Option #3. Option #2 would actually decrease the thoracic expansion of the chest wall on the right side. Option #4 is incorrect because there is no basis to make a judgment about the type of treatment.

9.5 ③ Option #3 is correct. If the UAP is providing a bath and client is incontinent, it would be an infection control violation to wear gloves when opening the door. The nurse does need to intervene due to the risk of this action and educate the UAP on infection control precautions. Options #1, #2, and #4 do not require the nurse to intervene since these nursing actions would be appropriate for this client.

I CAN HINT: Option #1 is a general answer and is not specific to the clinical situation in the stem of the question. Since the question asks "which of the actions should the nurse intervene with," "**SAFETY**" would be the priority observation. "*Infection Control Precautions*" is a great clinical decision making strategy, since this is one of the leading causes for client complications in the hospital. It is in the top 5 NCLEX® activities!

9.6 ③ Option #3 is the correct answer. These symptoms must be reported since they may be a result of a urinary tract infection and mandate further assessment and intervention. Options #1 is not a priority since this may be indicative of stress incontinence. Option #2 may be a result of osteoarthritis and is unfortunately expected with this condition. This definitely causes discomfort, but is not a priority over the possibility of an infection as in option #3. Option #4 would not be a priority since this HR is above 60 BPM.

9.7 ④ Option #4 is the correct answer. This clinical finding may be indicative of a complication with bleeding. Options # 1, #2, and #3 are expected findings following this procedure.

9.8 ② Option #2 is the correct answer. Clients with sickle cell crisis experience a blocking of the blood flow and causing cellular hypoxia from the sickle-shaped RBCs sticking to the capillary wall and each other. Copious amounts of oral or I.V. fluids are used to correct hypovolemia and prevent dehydration and further vessel occlusion. Starting this client's IV is imperative for the management of care. Option #1 is important to intervene with, but is not a priority over option #2. Option #3 is important to implement, but is not a priority over option #2. Option #4 is not a priority since surgery is not for 2 hours.

9.9 ① Option #1 is the correct answer. Option #1 measures the pressure on the right side of the heart. If the CVP is maintained, then the client will be adequately perfused and the urine output will increase. The vital signs and urine output are not problematic for a client who is only 1 hour post-op. If the client had been out of surgery for several hours, then the urine output would be more of a concern. Option #2 is not appropriate for this client. This medication may result in a lower blood pressure which could lead to a compromise in the cardiac perfusion of the client resulting in a lower urine output. Option #3 is not appropriate and may lead to more complications. Option #4 is not appropriate or necessary at the present time due to the post-op time frame.

9.10 ① Option #1 is the correct answer. This is the next priority to notify the physician since the signs indicate pulmonary edema.

Options #2 and #3 would increase fluids to the lungs. Option #4 is incorrect because the nurse should stay with the client for reassurance.

9.11 ② Option #2 is the correct answer. The client is presenting with hypoglycemia, and if client receives the insulin the symptoms will get worse. The nurse needs to intervene due to unsafe practice. Options #1, #3, and #4 all represent safe nursing practice.

9.12 ③ Option #3 is the correct answer. If a dressing becomes saturated or soiled, it is a priority to change the bandage. Bacteria grow well in a warm moist environment, and the nurse would need to change the bandage as soon as able. Option #1 is not relevant to the nurse's plan. Option #2 would require the nurse assess and treat the client's pain, but not change the dressing. Option #4 indicates that the client is ready; however, in prioritizing nursing care, the nurse must determine what task is to be completed first.

9.13 ① Option #1 is the correct answer. Airway is the priority. The client's clinical changes have occurred due to hypoxia. Providing oxygen will maintain the client until the provider of care can reintubate. Option #2 is incorrect since client has a pulse. Option #3 is incorrect since hypoxia is not secondary to hypovolemia. Option #4 is not a priority over the airway management.

9.14 ① Option #1 is the correct answer. The priority is to maintain moisture to prevent the wound from drying out and becoming necrotic prior to the client returning to surgery. Option #2 is not the priority for this clinical situation. Option #3 needs to be moist in order to be a correct answer. Option #4 needs to be continuous to be a correct answer.

9.15 ④ Option #4 would be done first.
      ⑤ Option #5 would be done second.
      ① Option #1 would be done third.
      ② Option #2 would be done fourth.
      ③ Option #3 would be done fifth.

9.16 ① Option #1 is correct answer. Battery failure will cause the pacemaker to be inoperable. The client may experience a heart block or the signs presented in the situation. Pacing spikes will not occur if the pacemaker is not firing. Options #2, #3, and #4 are incorrect.

9.17 ④ Option #4 is the correct answer. One of the most reliable physical findings of a deep vein thrombosis, a post-op complication, is edema of the affected leg. When discovered, a nurse should measure both legs at mid-thigh and mid-calf, so that the nurse's report to the provider of care is complete and accurate. Option #1 is incorrect because increased activity of the leg without concurrent treatment for deep vein thrombosis may actually dislodge the clot. Option #2 is incorrect because it does not address the immediate need of the client, and in renal failure and heart failure, edema is bilateral. Option #3 is incorrect because it does not address the immediate need of the client, and will not help to resolve the problem of a deep vein thrombosis.

9.18 ③ Option #3 is the correct answer. It is the safest for the client and will allow time to set up another pleur-evac. Option #1 is unsafe and could result in a mediastinal shift if the clamp is left on too long. The majority of physicians will request the chest tubes not be clamped. Option #2 is not a priority over option #3. Option #4 is incorrect for this clinical situation.

9.19 ② Option #2 is the correct. An air leak would not allow negative pressure to be reestablished and would hinder complete resolution of the pneumothorax. Therefore, partial atelectasis could be noted. Option #1 is an appropriate order for chest tubes. Option #3 does not hinder the chest tube functioning. Option #4 would be an expected finding. It would be important for the nurse to ensure tube patency.

9.20 ① Option #1 is the correct answer because stopping the infusion will decrease contractions and possibly remove uterine pressure on the fetus, which is a possible cause of the late deceleration. Option #2 may help the late deceleration, but is not a priority over option #1, and would be done after the oxytocin was stopped. Options #3 and #4 will have no influence and do not address the issue presented in the stem of the question which is the prolonged late decelerations and the oxytocin.

9.21 ③ Option #3 is the correct answer. When the low pressure alarm sounds, this usually indicates a leak. Options #1, #2 and #4 would result in a high pressure alarm.

9.22 ④ Option #4 is the correct answer. This will prevent alveoli collapse and assist the client in controlling the rate and depth of breathing. Option #1 is not correct. Confusion is most likely due to hypoxia versus electrolyte imbalance. There is nothing in the stem of the question to indicate the client is experiencing vomiting, diarrhea, etc. which would result in fluid and electrolyte imbalance. Option #2 is not a priority over option #4. While the temperature does need to be evaluated to determine a potential infection, the immediate concern is with the oxygenation, so the encouragement of pursed-lip breathing would be the priority. The temperature would then be evaluated. The confusion with an elderly client may be secondary to either hypoxia or sepsis. Option #3 is incorrect because client should receive low flow oxygen to prevent carbon dioxide narcosis.

9.23 ① Option #1 is the correct answer. Head of bed elevated at 60 – 90 degrees will displace the abdominal organs by gravity. Option #2 will cause the diaphragm to go against the abdominal organs. Option #3 is incorrect. The head of bed would only be elevated 15-30 degrees. Option #4 will result in problems breathing.

9.24 ③ Option #3 is the correct answer. This will prevent infection. Option #1 is incorrect. The inner cannula needs to be removed and cleaned 8 hours and PRN. Option #2 is incorrect. They may even need to be changed PRN or more frequently. The old

ties need to stay in place until the new ones are in place. Option #4 is incorrect since humidification is important to liquefy the secretions.

9.25 ③ Option #3 is the correct answer. This is a sign of angina which is what the client is experiencing. The elevated ST segment indicates an MI. Option #1 indicates hyperkalemia. Option #2 indicates hypokalemia. Option #4 indicates a heart block.

9.26 ④ Option #4 is the correct answer. Ketoacidosis which could result from insulin decrease and signs and symptoms may be polyuria, polydipsia, dry mucous membranes, nausea and vomiting, weight loss, hypotension, abdominal pain, shock, and coma. Option #1 is incorrect. These are signs of hypoglycemia from too much insulin. Option #2 is incorrect. These are signs of an infection. Option #3 is incorrect. These are signs of hyperglycemic hyperosmolar nonketotic coma. Other symptoms may be polyphagia, polyuria, polydipsia, glycosuria, changes in LOC, hypotension, and shock.

9.27 ③ Option #3 is the correct answer. Total parenteral nutrition (TPN), or hyperalimentation, has high glucose content. Therefore, it is important to monitor glucose levels. Options #1, #2, and #4 are not priorities over option #3 during the first 24 hours.

9.28 ① Option #1 is the correct answer since the medication is administered IV. Options #2, #3, and #4 are incorrect. Option #2, doing a complete assessment, is not necessary prior to administering this medication. Option #3 indicates the vital signs which includes more than the temperature. This is not necessary immediately prior to administering an IV antibiotic. Option #4 does not address the question which reads "prior to administering" and the answer reads "evaluates symptoms" as if the medication is already infusing.

9.29 ③ Option #3 is the correct answer. This will assist in preventing further atelectasis, and it can be measured. Options #1, #2, and #4 are not correct. Option #1 is incorrect because when compared to option #3 it cannot be measured. If option #3 was not included as an option, then option #1 would be correct. Option #2 is incorrect due to positioning. Option #4 is not a priority over option #3.

9.30 ④ Option #4 is a priority since the client could be bleeding or hypoxic. Options #1, #2, and #3 are incorrect for this clinical situation.

9.31 ④ Option #4 is correct in preventing complications with pneumonia. Option #1 is not within the scope of practice for the nurse to provide education on the surgical procedure. The nurse is responsible for the teaching and implementation of the nursing care and verifying the consent is on the chart. The physician is responsible for information regarding the surgical procedure. Option #2 is not appropriate. Option #3 is not a priority over #4.

9.32 ① Option #1 is the correct answer. Client is presenting with hypoglycemia. Giving a fast acting sugar and protein would be most appropriate for this client. Option #2 is not appropriate for these symptoms of hypoglycemia. Option #3 is not a priority. Option #4 is not necessary. Action is necessary versus spending time notifying provider of care.

9.33 ② Option #2 may be septic and needs to be further evaluated. Options #1, #3, and #4 are not a priority to #2.

9.34 ③ Option #3 is a priority. Always establish unresponsiveness prior to initiating the other options.

9.35 ③ Option #3 is the correct answer. A client with COPD can have chronically low oxygen saturation, and is not symptomatic from a low level. The symptoms of hypoxia in a client with COPD are anxiety and agitation, as the oxygen level is always low; the onset of these symptoms (hypoxia) is of greatest concern. The client suffers from COPD, which would explain options #1 and #4. The low oxygen level and the shortness of breath on exertion are common findings in the client with COPD. Option #2 is explained by the diabetes, and this is not a critical value.

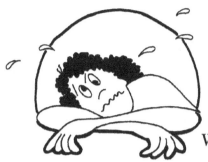 *Way to go! Take a break before taking the post-tests.*

Passion is energy. Feel the power that comes from focusing on what excites you.
—Oprah Winfrey

✔ **Clarification of this test ...**

This post-test and the bonus post-test are comprehensive, integrated exams and are comparable to the pre-test. The first 50 questions on this test reflect the pre-test and the following questions are new. We suggest you complete the other chapters prior to taking the post-tests.

10.1 What task can be delegated to the UAP?

① Obtain a dietary history from a client diagnosed with anorexia.

② Assist a client with diabetes who is learning how to perform a glucometer check.

③ Assess the judgment of a client admitted with a head injury secondary to a fall.

④ Obtain a stool specimen from a client with diarrhea secondary to Salmonella.

10.2 What is the priority of care for a 16-year-old married client who is to have a Caesarean section to deliver a baby?

① Notify the legal guardians to sign the surgical consent.

② Ask the spouse to sign the surgical consent since the client is 16 years old.

③ Ask the 16-year-old client to sign the consent.

④ Delay the medical intervention until the parent arrives to the hospital.

10.3 What is the priority of care for an older adult client who is post-op following a hip replacement?

① Review the importance for client to lift leg upward from a lying position.

② Encourage client to elevate the knee when sitting.

③ Keep abductor pillow in place while client is in bed.

④ Review exercises with client on how to flex hip 90 degrees or more to prevent stiffness.

10.4 Which of these statements about hepatitis A indicates the LPN understood the health promotion information that was given to a group of nurses who are in orientation for Home Health Nursing?

① "Standard precautions are the appropriate type of infection precautions."

② "Nurses should wear gloves and a gown when in contact with the client."

③ "Nurses should wear gloves, gown, and a mask when in contact with client."

④ "Hepatitis A is transmitted by blood and airborne droplets, so airborne precautions should be followed."

10.5 Which of these actions by an unlicensed assistive personnel (UAP) when working with a post-CVA client who has a right-sided paralysis would require intervention by the LPN?

① The UAP takes the blood pressure on the left arm.
② The UAP places the wheelchair on the right side of the bed when getting out of bed.
③ The UAP provides high-top tennis shoes for the client to prevent foot drop.
④ The UAP approaches the client on the unaffected when approaching the bedside.

10.6 An 85-year-old client cannot swallow the antibiotic tablet. Which is the priority action?

① Crush the tablets, dissolve in milk, and allow the client to swallow them.
② Notify the healthcare provider for a different order.
③ Ask the pharmacist if liquid is available in this medication.
④ Ask family members to coax the client to swallow the tablets.

10.7 The client diagnosed with congestive heart failure wakes in the middle of the night gasping and saying "I can't breathe!" Which would be the priority nursing action?

① Place the client in the supine position and suction airway.
② Elevate the head of the bed.
③ Administer oxygen per protocol at 4L/minute.
④ Assess the client's lung sounds.

10.8 The client diagnosed with diabetes mellitus has been prescribed a Methyl Prednisolone Dose Pack. What would be most important for the nurse to monitor for the client taking this drug?

① Serum glucose.
② Hemoglobin.
③ Stools for occult blood.
④ Vital Signs.

10.9 The client's admitting vital signs as recorded by the registered nurse were documented as P–80, R–20, BP–170/90. Half hour later the vital signs are P–82, R– 2, BP–190/100. What would be the priority nursing action?

① Notify the Charge RN of the change in vital signs.
② Wait 15 minutes and retake the BP.
③ Document the findings.
④ Ask the client if he salted his lunch.

10.10 During the orientation session for new LPNs / LVNs, the instructor reviewed calcium channel blockers. During the clinical evaluation on the medical unit, the LPN has a client that just received the first dose of Norvasc (amlodipine) an hour ago. Which of these assessments indicate the LPN understands how to evaluate the client response to this medication?

① Respiratory rate
② Reflexes
③ Temperature
④ Blood pressure

10.11 Which of these clients should the nurse assess immediately after shift report?

① A client complaining of dizziness after getting out of bed quickly.
② A client who just stopped talking and is slumped over in bed.
③ A client with a blood pressure of 110/76 and it was 120/84 two hours earlier.
④ A client with a heart rate of 90 BPM.

10.12 What would be the priority nursing action for a client diagnosed with diabetes mellitus who presents with confusion, shaking, and diaphoresis?

① Assess vital signs.
② Administer insulin as ordered.
③ Provide client with a glass of milk.
④ Notify the HCP.

10.13 A client on renal dialysis taking warfarin (Coumadin) has decided to take Gingko Biloba for memory loss. What is the priority action?

① Take the Gingko from the client and flush it down the toilet.

② Confirm that the Gingko has been successfully used by client with decreased memory loss.

③ Inform the RN of this client decision.

④ Explain that both drugs administered together may cause bleeding tendencies.

10.14 The client's medical record indicates that a client is allergic to penicillin. There is a new order to administer acyclovir (Zovirax). Which nursing action would be the priority?

① Hold the acyclovir (Zovirax) as there is an incompatibility with penicillin.

② Notify the HCP of the allergy to penicillin.

③ Assess the client's BUN and creatinine prior to administering the drug.

④ Assess the client's temperature prior to administering the medication.

10.15 The mother of a 21-year-old asks the Emergency Department nurse to identify the admitting diagnosis for her son. Which action is most important?

① Advise the mother of the admitting diagnosis and ask for the name of the family provider.

② Ask the RN to speak to the mother.

③ Tell the mother that her son is of age and the diagnosis cannot be revealed to her.

④ Inform the mother that confidentiality laws prevent the release of information.

10.16 Which of the following should be included in the process for changing a dressing on a newborn? *Select all that apply.*

① Wash hands thoroughly and apply sterile gloves.

② Utilize sterile bandaging and secure with paper tape.

③ Teach the care giver the process for changing the bandage.

④ Dispose of the old bandage in an appropriate receptacle.

⑤ Document the procedure as being a "clean dressing change."

10.17 An elderly client, who resides in an assisted living facility, has been experiencing some delusions in the lunch room and is asking for the "before meal pill." The armband is lost. What would be the most appropriate action prior to administering the medication?

① Ask the client to state name and administer the medication.

② Ask the client's roommate for the name prior to administering medication and replace the armband.

③ Ask the UAP for the name of the client.

④ Determine the client's identification by checking the chart for a photograph.

10.18 What is the priority nursing action for a post operative client who has been admitted with Clostridium Difficile?

① Clean hands with alcohol antiseptic hand wash.

② Place client in private room and wear gloves and gown during nursing care.

③ Place client in a room with a client who has MRSA.

④ Wear gloves and mask when in the client's room.

10.19 A five-foot tall client that weighs 179 pounds is to receive an I.M. injection of Bicillin. Which size needle should be selected for use?

① 20 gauge, 3 inch needle.

② 21 gauge, 1 to 1½ inch needle.

③ 25 gauge, 1 to 1½ inch needle.

④ 25 gauge 5/8 inch needle.

10.20 A 32-year-old pregnant client reporting episodes of rapid breathing, air hunger and tingling has an oxygen saturation reading of 97%. Which would be the appropriate nursing actions? *Select all that apply.*

① Assist the client to a high-Fowler's position.
② Reassess the client's O$_2$ saturation reading.
③ Administer oxygen @ 4L /minute per protocol.
④ Turn the client to the left side and apply oxygen @ 1L/minute per protocol.
⑤ Notify the healthcare provider of the assessment and nursing actions.

10.21 A 62-year-old client, who is second day post-operative hip replacement, has an order to ambulate in the hall. The client expresses fear of getting out of the bed. What would be the appropriate nursing actions? *Select all that apply.*

① Ask an additional staff member to assist with the ambulation.
② Ask a family member to walk beside the client with a wheelchair in case this is needed.
③ Place a safety belt on the client that can be used to steady the walk.
④ Place a safety belt on both staff members for client to reach if needed.
⑤ Explain to the client the time and distance of the walk.

10.22 What is the priority of care for any client who experiences a seizure?

① Maintain a patent airway for the client.
② Assess vital signs prior to further action.
③ Ask the client if they can hear you.
④ Lower the client to the floor and wait for the seizure to be complete.

10.23 The daughter of a client who is in a nursing home reports that her mother has been beaten and has the bruises to prove it. Which actions should be taken? *Select all that apply.*

① Assess the client's bruises and ask her how she got them.
② Read the chart to determine if there are any recorded accident reports.
③ Speak to staff caring for the client and assess their reports.
④ File an incident report as reported by the daughter.
⑤ Call the police to report a possible assault and battery.

10.24 The client is to receive haloperidol (Haldol) 2mg injectable which is provided in 5mg/mL. How many mLs will be administered to this client? **Fill in the blank.**
_____mLs

10.25 In planning the care of a client with an acute episode of Meniere's syndrome, the client should be taught which of the following?

① Adding salt to food.
② Avoiding sudden motion of the head.
③ Placing client in room closest to nurses' station.
④ Encouraging client to be up walking in hall.

10.26 Which technique is best for obtaining a urine specimen for a culture and sensitivity from a client with an existing indwelling catheter?

① Clean the drain of the collecting bag with an antiseptic before filling the specimen container.
② Obtain the specimen from the drainage bag in the morning.
③ Using a sterile syringe with a small gauge needle, aspirate urine from the catheter port.
④ If the catheter has been in place for 48 hours, replace it before obtaining the specimen.

10.27 Which procedure indicates the nurse understands how to safely administer the DPT immunization to a 6-month-old child? The nurse administers the DPT:

   ① By mouth in three divided doses.

   ② As an IM injection into the gluteus maximus.

   ③ As an injection into the vastus lateralis.

   ④ As a deep Z track injection into the deltoid.

10.28 1000 ml 5% Dextrose in 0.45 Saline is to be administered IV over 8 hours using an infusion pump for an adult client. What is the correct rate setting on the IV pump? **Fill in the blank.** _____ mL / hour.

10.29 To promote safety, the nurse would implement which action in obtaining a blood specimen from a client who has been diagnosed with hepatitis B?

   ① Clean area with antiseptic solution.

   ② Wear a pair of clean gloves.

   ③ Apply pressure to site for 5 seconds.

   ④ Recap needle to avoid carrying exposed needle.

10.30 Organize these steps in chronological order with #1 being the first step for a client who is having a nasogastric tube removal.

   ① Assist the client into a semi-Fowler's position.

   ② Ask client to hold breath.

   ③ Assess bowel function by auscultation for peristalsis.

   ④ Flush tube with 10 ml of normal saline.

   ⑤ Withdraw the tube gently and steadily.

   ⑥ Monitor client for nausea, vomiting.

10.31 Which side effect of Trimethoprim-sulfamethoxazole (Bactrim) should the nurse instruct the client to report while taking this medication?

   ① Hypotonia.

   ② Loss of hearing.

   ③ Hypotension.

   ④ Urticaria.

10.32 Following an abdominal hysterectomy, which action would be a priority in preventing thrombophlebitis?

   ① Encourage support by using knee gatch.

   ② Decrease the fluid intake.

   ③ Encourage turning, coughing, and deep breathing every 2 hours.

   ④ Encourage active leg exercises and ambulation.

10.33 Following the death of a female client who is Muslim, the nurse should plan on providing the family with:

   ① A private room to gather the family for grieving.

   ② A Muslim wrap, preferably white, for the body.

   ③ Post-mortem care of the body by a female nurse.

   ④ Immediate referral to a crematory.

10.34 A 72-year-old client has an order for digoxin (Lanoxin) 0.25 mg po in the morning. The nurse reviews the following information: apical pulse = 68 BPM, respirations = 16/min., plasma digoxin level = 2.2 ng/mL. Based on this assessment, which nursing action is appropriate?

   ① Give the medication on time.

   ② Withhold the medication and notify the healthcare provider.

   ③ Administer epinephrine 1:1000 stat.

   ④ Check the client's blood pressure.

10.35 Which of these psychiatric clients should be evaluated first?

   ① Depressed client sitting on the floor rocking back and forth.

   ② Bipolar client pacing and clenching fist.

   ③ Psychotic client who is having a delusion that she is the Queen of England.

   ④ Schizophrenic client laughing and waving hands up in the air.

10.36 Which communication technique would be appropriate for a nurse to implement when caring for a client who has a hearing loss?

① Irrigate the ear with warm water to remove any wax obstruction.
② Always touch the client prior to speaking to him.
③ Encourage the client to purchase a hearing aid.
④ Stand in front of him and speak clearly and slowly.

10.37 What would be a priority in establishing a bladder retraining program?

① Provide a flexible schedule for the client to decrease anxiety.
② Schedule toileting on a planned time schedule.
③ Teach client intermittent self-catheterization.
④ Perform the Crede maneuver tid.

10.38 What is the correct procedure for obtaining a throat culture from a client with pharyngitis?

① Quickly rub a cotton swab over both tonsil and posterior pharynx areas.
② Obtain a sputum container for the client to use.
③ Swab the pharynx following irrigation with warm saline.
④ Hyperextend the client's head and neck for the procedure.

10.39 Which assessment would be most important for monitoring a client's state of hydration?

① Daily weights.
② I & O.
③ Skin tugor.
④ Characteristic of lips and mucous membranes.

10.40 A client discharged with sublingual nitroglycerin (Nitrostat) should be taught to:

① Take the medications 5 minutes after the pain has started.
② Stop taking the medication if a burning sensation is present.

③ Take the medication on an empty stomach.
④ Avoid abrupt changes in posture.

10.41 What is the priority nursing action prior to administering medications through a nasogastric tube?

① Consult a drug book regarding the recommendations for crushing each medication.
② Verify placement of the nasogastric tube in the abdomen through aspiration of gastric content.
③ Calculate the amount of water needed to dissolve each medication.
④ Clean out the pill crushers to get rid of any residue.

10.42 The psychiatric nurse is administering a depressed client doxepin hydrochloride (Sinequan) 75 mg po TID. This nurse should recommend a change in the client's therapy if which response occurs? The client:

① Refuses to speak and sits quietly in the room.
② Becomes excitable and develops tremors.
③ Refuses to eat breakfast.
④ Sleeps 18 hours a day.

10.43 Which nursing approach would be most appropriate to use while administering an oral medication to a 4-month-old child?

① Place medication in 45 mL of formula.
② Place medication in an empty nipple.
③ Place medication in a full bottle of formula.
④ Place in supine position and administer medication using a syringe.

10.44 Which clinical finding would be most appropriate for the LPN to report to the RN regarding the client taking furosemide (Lasix)?

① A weight loss of two pounds.
② Blood pressure change from 160/98 to 141/90.
③ An increase in urinary frequency.
④ A ringing in the ears.

10.45 Which sequence is correct when providing care for a client immediately prior to surgery?

① Administer preoperative medication, client signs operative permit, determine vital signs.
② Check operative permit for signature, advise the client to remain in bed, administer preoperative medication.
③ Remove client's dentures, administer preoperative medication, client empties bladder.
④ Verify client has been NPO. Client empties bladder, family leaves room.

10.46 A permanent demand pacemaker set at a rate of 72 beats per minute is implanted in a client for persistent third degree block. Which nursing assessment would indicate a pacemaker dysfunction?

① Pulse rate of 88 and irregular.
② Apical pulse rate regular at 68.
③ Blood pressure of 110/88 and pulse 78.
④ Tenderness at site of pacemaker implant.

10.47 A 24-year-old client who is 2 hours post-delivery complains of nausea, being cold, and "feeling funny." Vital signs indicate a BP–80/40, Pulse–120 beats per minute, Respirations–26 per minute. Which nursing action would be a priority?

① Assess for bleeding.
② Place in Trendelenberg position.
③ Contact the healthcare provider.
④ Administer PRN pain medication.

10.48 To complete an assessment of cranial nerve eleven, the client will be asked to:

① Move tongue.
② Identify a smell.
③ Read a Snellen chart.
④ Shrug both shoulders.

10.49 A round reddened quarter sized area is assessed on a bedridden client's coccyx area during the morning assessment. Which actions should be taken to improve skin integrity? *Select all that apply.*

① Clean and dry the area carefully.
② Place the client on a "turn every 2 hour" plan.
③ Document the size, induration and skin condition.
④ Notify the provider for treatment options.
⑤ Place the client on appropriate isolation program.

10.50 In receiving morning report, the night nurse relates that the nurse on the previous shift forgot to sign off one of the charts; therefore, a space of a few lines was left for the nurse when returns to work. Which is the most appropriate action?

① Notify the supervisor prior to the night nurse leaving the unit.
② Call the nurse who forgot to chart to come in today to complete the chart.
③ Chart as usual leaving the blank space for the off duty nurse.
④ Notify the healthcare provider for direction.

10.51 The client has an order for 150 mL /hour of IV Ringer's lactate. The IV administration set delivers 10 gtts/mL. At what rate should the nurse set the infusion? **Fill in the blank**. _____ gtts / minute

10.52 A fire develops in the unit at a long term care facility. The fire department is on the way, but due to thick smoke, the unit must be evacuated. Which client should the nurse evacuate first?

① A client who had a Cesarean section 45 minutes ago.
② A 30-year-old client who had an appendectomy 6 hours ago.
③ An 84-year-old client recovering from pneumonia.
④ An elderly client with COPD and is being maintained on IV fluids.

10.53 An adult client is to receive heparin sodium (Heparin) 5,000 units subcutaneously. Which technique indicates the nurse understood the information learned in orientation regarding the appropriate technique for the administration of this drug? The LPN:

① Gently massages the injection site.
② Administers the drug without aspirating.
③ Uses a one inch 18–20 gauge needle.
④ Administers the drug in the deltoid muscle.

10.54 List in chronological order how the nurse should put on the personal protection equipment?

① Gloves
② Gown
③ Goggles or face shield
④ Mask or respirator

10.55 The LPN is working for a home healthcare agency. Which finding, if observed, should be reported by the nurse? A client

① with an infected wound who allows cats to eat off the table.
② receiving intermittent oxygen therapy who has a spouse that smokes in the home.
③ with diabetes who has a bowl of candy sitting on the coffee table.
④ with COPD who sleeps in a recliner instead of a bed.

10.56 Which documentation on an incident report is correct? The client is:

① found lying on floor after attempting to get out of bed. Call light on bed.
② found lying in the prone position, 3 feet from bed. Side rails up x2; call light at bedside.
③ attempting to get out of bed and fell. Found lying prone; call light on bed.
④ found lying prone position, approximately 5 feet from bed. Side rails up x2; call light at bedside.

10.57 A young child is newly diagnosed with type 1 diabetes mellitus. While reinforcing the discharge teaching with the parent, the mother states, "I have three other children and don't know how I am going to make all these special meals." What action made by the LPN would be beneficial to this family?

① Reassure the mother that you will take care of this situation.
② Consult with the RN for the possible need for a referral to a nutritionist.
③ Inform the charge nurse of the parent's anxiety regarding caring for the child at home.
④ Develop a dietary menu for the family to follow.

10.58 While at work, the LPN observes two UAPs in a heated argument in the hallway. What would be the most effective way to handle this situation?

① Quietly reprimand the UAPs and tell them to go back to work.
② Order the UAPs to leave the unit immediately.
③ Escort the UAPs to the office and file misconduct reports.
④ Escort the UAPs to a private area and determine the source of the conflict.

10.59 What information would be a priority to include in the orientation program for a group of nurses who will be providing care for clients being discharged from the cardiac unit following cardiac valve replacements? Prior to any dental surgery, the client should:

① Remain NPO.
② Check with the physician.
③ Start a new course of Heparin.
④ Discuss the need with the dentist to take a prescribed course of antibiotics.

10.60 A physician is meeting with a client regarding an upcoming procedure. When the physician comes out of the room he states, "I left the consent in the room for the client to sign. Can you sign as a witness?" When the nurse enters the room, the consent form is already signed. What should the nurse do?

① Inform the physician the consent was signed.
② Sign as the witness on the consent.
③ Sign as the witness and have the client
④ Obtain a new consent form.

10.61 Which of these nursing actions from the UAP would require immediate intervention from the nurse for a client presenting with heart failure from the recent diagnosis of infective endocarditis?

① The UAP uses a soft tooth brush during oral hygiene.
② The UAP encourages frequent ambulation in the hall during the day.
③ The UAP provides client with a snack when the nurse administers the Indomethacin (Indocin).
④ The UAP reports to the nurse the client's HR has increased from 68 BPM to 88 BPM.

10.62 Which interventions are appropriate for providing care for a client with Clostridium Difficile? *Select all that apply.*

① Share room with a client who has MRSA.
② Clean hands with alcohol after care.
③ Place mask on before going into room.
④ Place gown on when in client contact.
⑤ Place gloves on when in client contact.

10.63 Which nursing action would be most appropriate in helping a client, who is elderly and depressed, complete activities of daily living?

① Medicate client before activities are done.

② Assist client with grooming activities, so it does not take so long.
③ Develop a written schedule of activities, allowing extra time.
④ Provide forceful direction to keep the client focused.

10.64 Which information for a client with a tracheostomy would be most important to include in the shift report?

① SaO_2–96%, HR–80 BPM, RR–22/min.
② Suctioned thin, white secretions from tracheostomy.
③ Skin surrounding tracheostomy is red, increased Temp. from 97.8 to 99.9 degrees F.
④ Breath sounds with some adventitious sounds prior to suctioning.

10.65 Which of these nursing actions should be implemented by the LPN / LVN prior to admitting a client with the diagnosis of seizure disorder?

① Complete the admission assessment.
② Develop the plan of care for this client and share with UAP.
③ Place a padded tongue depressor at bedside.
④ Set up suction and oxygen equipment at the bedside.

10.66 Which of these interventions delegated to the LPN, who is providing care for a client with a pulmonary embolus (PE), indicate the new graduate understands the scope of practice for the LPN / LVN?

① Auscultate breath sounds for crackles.
② Assess new complaints of chest pain.
③ Monitor labs to assist with interpreting necessary oxygen changes.
④ Develop discharge plan.

10.67 Which assessment finding would be most important to report to provider of care for a client who has been discharged from the hospital after being in the hospital for 3 days with a left leg deep vein thrombosis (DVT) and a pulmonary embolism and is taking enoxaparin (Lovenox) 80 mg subcutaneously every 12 hours?

① The left calf is warm to touch and is larger than the right.
② The client has an ecchymotic area on leg.
③ The client reports not being able to have a pTT drawn.
④ The client is unable to remember her daughter's name.

10.68 Which nursing intervention indicates the LPN / LVN understands how to provide care for a client who is intubated, mechanically ventilated, and the "high pressure alarm" sounds? The nurse:

① Disables alarm and calls provider of care for an order for an arterial blood gas.
② Provides oxygen with an ambu bag and notifies provider of care.
③ Silences the alarm and notifies provider of care.
④ Suctions client and evaluates pulse oximeter.

10.69 Which of these would be the most appropriate to assign to the LPN? *Select all that apply.* A client who:

① has the diagnosis of myasthenia gravis.
② is receiving chemotherapy.
③ is a new admission with chest pain.
④ is being discharged and needs new diabetic teaching.
⑤ is in Buck's traction.

10.70 After receiving report from the RN, which of the following clients should the LPN/LVN see first? A client with acute respiratory failure who:

① Has a BP 120/80, HR–86 BPM, RR–20/min.
② Has a temperature of 99.2 degrees F from 98.4 degrees F.
③ Is restless, 0800 – HR–88 BPM, 0900 HR–100 BPM, pH–7.33, pCO_2–47 mm Hg.
④ Is resting, 0800 – RR–20/min, 0900 – RR–26/min, pH–7.34, pCO_2– 46.

10.71 The client has an order for a blood transfusion to be infused in over 4 hours. Which of these nursing actions is most appropriate for preparing and/or monitoring the transfusion? *Select all that apply.*

① Verify the identity of the client.
② Verify the blood with another nurse prior to hanging.
③ Use a #20 gauge needle for venous access for transfusion.
④ Assess the client's skin.
⑤ Stop the transfusion if the client exhibits difficulty in breathing.

10.72 Which of these statements would be most appropriate for a client with a spinal cord injury who states, "I am worthless now that I cannot move any part of my body"?

① "You should be happy to be alive!"
② "Why do you feel this way; you have so much to be thankful for."
③ "Do not lose hope; they are developing new techniques daily that may help in future."
④ "You sound like you have no hope."

10.73 Which of these assessments would be most important to report to HCP for the wife of a client who is a spinal cord injury client with a C_4 fracture?

① The wife indicates to the nurse that she may be in need of counseling to help her cope with her current situation.

② The wife has elicited the support of her family and friends in helping to provide care for her husband after discharge.

③ The wife has lost 10 lbs. since the accident, and shares with the nurse that her feelings of hopelessness about her future have resulted in her inability to sleep at night.

④ The wife reports that she is going to bed 1 hour earlier to get her needed rest to assist in handling the current situation of her husband.

10.74 The client has lost her appetite and the nurse learns that her daughter has recently died. Which of these is the priority nursing care?

① Call for an order for an IV to provided nutrition.

② Ask the client to talk about her daughter to you.

③ Call for an antidepressant order.

④ Explain that you know other people who have lost a loved one and they get over it.

10.75 The most important action to take prior to administering promethazine hydrochloride (Phenergan) IV would be to check:

① The client's blood pressure.

② The client's TPR.

③ Time the last analgesic was administered.

④ The patency of the vein.

10.76 While the nurse is irrigating an 86-year-old client's ear to remove cerumen, the client comments that he is getting dizzy. Which nursing actions are appropriate? *Select all that apply.*

① Stop the procedure immediately.

② Warm the irrigant and resume the procedure.

③ Monitor for increased intracranial pressure.

④ Notify the provider immediately.

⑤ Explore the canal with a cotton applicator.

10.77 The most important information for the nurse to obtain prior to a computerized axial tomography (CAT) scan concerns:

① problems with being in closed spaces.

② allergies to aspirin.

③ intact swallow and gag reflex.

④ full range of motion of all extremities.

10.78 Which reflex would be abnormal to observe in a 6-month-old child?

① Presence of a positive Babinski reflex.

② Extrusion reflex occurs when feeding.

③ Able to voluntarily grasp objects.

④ Rolls from abdomen to back at will.

10.79 Which observation indicates the client has an understanding of appropriate crutch walking?

① Weight bearing is under the arm on the axillary area.

② The crutches are placed about 18–20 inches in from of client with each step.

③ The weight of the body is being transferred to the hands and arms.

④ Leather-soled shoes are worn to increase the smooth motion across the floor.

10.80 Before administering the MMR (Measles, Mumps and Rubella) vaccine to a 15-month-old toddler, the nurse should check with the mother regarding: *Select all that apply.*

① A family history reaction to immunizations.

② Allergies to eggs or neomycin.

③ Allergies in siblings to medications.

④ Diarrhea without temperature in this toddler within the last week.

⑤ Determine if this immunization is age appropriate.

10.81 Which is the highest priority when inserting an indwelling urinary catheter?

① Aseptic technique.
② Taping the catheter to the leg.
③ Determining an allergy to latex.
④ Instilling water into the balloon.

10.82 The client has asked for pain medication following abdominal surgery. The nursing priority includes:

① Asking the client to determine the amount of pain on a scale of 1 to 10.
② Asking the client's significant other if the pain is worse than it was an hour ago.
③ Determine the last time the client had the pain medication.
④ Identify client allergies.

10.83 During the new born assessment, the nurse is evaluating the rooting reflex. Locate where the nurse would stroke to elicit this response.

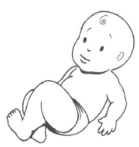

10.84 Which schedule would be most appropriate to recommend to a pre-menopausal woman regarding a self breast examination?

① One week prior to the menstrual period.
② One week after the menstrual period.
③ During every shower.
④ The same day once per month.

10.85 The provider should be notified about which assessment of a mother during her third trimester of pregnancy?

① Epigastric pain.
② Shortness of breath.
③ Increase in rectal pressure.
④ A total weight gain of 33 pounds.

10.86 Which clinical finding would be most important to report to the healthcare provider (HCP) for a client, who is post-op craniotomy, and is complaining of thirst and fatigue?

① Output of 6 L in 24 hours with a specific gravity of 1.000.
② Client refuses to lie on side of incision site.
③ Fluid intake over past 24 hours has been 2800 mL.
④ Specific gravity is 1.030 and urine is concentrated.

10.87 After assessing client's eating habits, which foods would the nurse recommend to the client on a low-residue diet? *Select all that apply.*

① Baked Chicken
② Rice
③ Plain Jell-O
④ Milk
⑤ Creamed chicken soup

10.88 During report, the nurse indicates that the client's nasogastric (NG) tube stopped draining over the last hour. Prior to that, it was draining 100 mL of fluid q 2 hr. Which plan would be priority?

① Remove the old tube and insert a new one.
② Reposition the tube to promote drainage.
③ Ask the provider for an order for a chest x-ray to determine accurate tube placement.
④ Force 50 mL of normal saline down the tube to irrigate it open.

10.89 Forty-five minutes after receiving 10 units of Humalog insulin, the client presents with diaphoresis, pale in color, and tachycardia. Which would be the priority nursing action?

① Call the RN supervisor.
② Offer the client milk and crackers.
③ Administer glucagon per protocol.
④ Call the lab for a stat blood glucose level.

I CAN Publishing®, INC.

10.90 A 21-year-female has just been told by the surgeon that her biopsy results indicate breast cancer. What would be the most appropriate nursing action?

① Ask the client if she has questions.
② Encourage the client to talk about her feelings.
③ Leave the client alone, so she can think.
④ Call the chaplain for the client.

10.91 Which nursing action indicates a need for further teaching regarding hand hygiene?

① Washes hands with soap and water when soiled after client care.
② Never reuses disposable gloves while providing care for client.
③ Uses alcohol hand sanitizers when hands are not visibly soiled.
④ Uses soap and water to clean under artificial nails.

10.92 Which of these changes on the cardiac monitor strip would occur for a client, in the assisted living facility, presenting with chest pain causing the LPN/LVN to suspect angina?

① Spiked T waves.
② Elevation in the ST segment.
③ Depressed ST segment.
④ Prolonged PR interval.

10.93 What information would be most important to share with next shift and the healthcare provider (HCP) for a client with a spinal cord injury who was placed in fixed skeletal traction with a Halo fixation device 2 weeks ago?

① "The wrench needed to release the rods from the vest is taped to front of vest."
② "The body is being maintained in appropriate alignment."
③ "The Halo insertion sites have been cleaned per hospital protocol."
④ "The Halo insertion sites are inflamed and swollen."

10.94 Which method is the best for the nurse to evaluate the effectiveness of tracheal suctioning?

① Assess vital signs.
② Auscultate the chest for change or clearing of adventitious breath sounds.
③ Consult with respiratory therapist to determine effectiveness.
④ Note subjective data such as, "My breathing is much improved now."

10.95 Two hours after a cardiac catheterization, the client begins to bleed from the femoral insertion site. Which nursing intervention would be most appropriate?

① Apply manual pressure and notify the provider of care.
② Assess pedal pulses and apply a sandbag.
③ Elevate the head of bed 40 degrees and apply an ice pack.
④ Place the client in Trendelenburg immediately.

SENDING LOVE
Since we're unable to meet,
I thought it would be neat,
to send something to keep,
to show my love is deep.
—MARGARET S. WRIGHT (1914–2003)
(Sylvia's mom)

CATEGORY ANALYSIS – PRE-TEST

1. Coordinated Care
2. Coordinated Care
3. Basic Care and Comfort
4. Safety & Infection Control
5. Safety & Infection Control
6. Pharmacological Therapies
7. Physiological Adaptation
8. Pharmacological Therapies
9. Reduction of Risk Potential
10. Pharmacological Therapies
11. Physiological Adaptation
12. Physiological Adaptation
13. Pharmacological Therapies
14. Pharmacological Therapies
15. Coordinated Care
16. Safety & Infection Control
17. Safety & Infection Control
18. Safety & Infection Control
19. Pharmacological Therapies
20. Physiological Adaptation
21. Safety & Infection Control
22. Reduction of Risk Potential
23. Coordinated Care
24. Pharmacological Therapies
25. Safety & Infection Control
26. Reduction of Risk Potential
27. Pharmacological Therapies
28. Pharmacological Therapies
29. Safety & Infection Control
30. Reduction of Risk Potential
31. Health Promotion
32. Basic Care and Comfort

33. Psychosocial Integrity
34. Physiological Adaptation
35. Psychosocial Integrity
36. Basic Care and Comfort
37. Basic Care and Comfort
38. Reduction of Risk Potential
39. Basic Care and Comfort
40. Health Promotion
41. Reduction of Risk Potential
42. Pharmacological Therapies
43. Health Promotion
44. Coordinated Care
45. Coordinated Care
46. Physiological Adaptation
47. Reduction of Risk Potential
48. Reduction of Risk Potential
49. Basic Care and Comfort
50. Coordinated Care
51. Pharmacological Therapies
52. Safety & Infection Control
53. Coordinated Care
54. Safety & Infection Control
55. Safety & Infection Control
56. Safety & Infection Control
57. Health Promotion
58. Coordinated Care
59. Coordinated Care
60. Coordinated Care
61. Coordinated Care
62. Safety & Infection Control
63. Psychosocial Integrity
64. Coordinated Care

65. Reduction of Risk Potential
66. Coordinated Care
67. Pharmacological Therapies
68. Physiological Adaptation
69. Coordinated Care
70. Coordinated Care
71. Pharmacological Therapies
72. Psychosocial Integrity
73. Psychosocial Integrity
74. Psychosocial Integrity
75. Pharmacological Therapies
76. Health Promotion
77. Reduction of Risk Potential
78. Health Promotion
79. Basic Care and Comfort
80. Health Promotion
81. Safety & Infection Control
82. Basic Care and Comfort
83. Health Promotion
84. Health Promotion
85. Reduction of Risk Potential
86. Basic Care and Comfort
87. Basic Care and Comfort
88. Reduction of Risk Potential
89. Physiological Adaptation
90. Psychosocial Integrity
91. Safety & Infection Control
92. Physiological Adaptation
93. Physiological Adaptation
94. Reduction of Risk Potential
95. Reduction of Risk Potential

DIRECTIONS

1. Determine questions missed by checking answers.
2. Write the number of the questions missed across the top line marked "item missed."
3. Check category analysis page to determine category of question.
4. Put a check mark under item missed and beside content.
5. Count check marks in each row and write the number in totals column.
6. Use this information to:
   • identify areas for further study.
   • determine which content test to take next.

We recommend studying content where most items are missed—then taking that content test.

Number of the Questions Incorrectly Answered

Pret-est	Items Missed																																			Totals
C Coordinated Care																																				
O Safety and Infection Control																																				
N Health Promotion and Maintenance																																				
T Psychosocial Integrity																																				
E Physiological Integrity: Physiological Adaptation																																				
N Physiological Integrity: Reduction of Risk																																				
T Physiological Integrity: Basic Care and Comfort																																				
Physiological Integrity: Pharmacological Therapies																																				

I CAN Publishing®, INC.

NOTES

ANSWERS & RATIONALES

10.1 ④ Option #4 is correct. The key to answering this question correctly is to understand the scope of practice for the UAP. The UAP is able to perform tasks that are routine and are similar in the steps each time the task is implemented. Refer to I CAN HINT for an easy way to remember the scope of practice for the UAP. Option #1 is incorrect since the UAP would need to assess this from the client and need to use specific communication principles in order to facilitate the dietary history. Initiating a history on the client is not within the scope of practice for the UAP. Option #2 is incorrect since the client is learning how to perform the task. If the client was not learning and this was a routine task then this would be acceptable for the UAP as an assignment. Option #3 is incorrect since the client requires an assessment and a clinical decision requiring clinical judgment are definitely not within the scope of practice for the UAP.

 I CAN HINT: Tasks to be delegated to the UAP can be remembered by reviewing "BART."

Baths (routine and uncomplicated)

Ambulation

Routine tasks

Tasks that do not require critical thinking/ clinical decision making

10.2 ③ Option #3 is correct. A minor who is lawfully married and any competent individual 18 or older can sign a surgical consent. Other options are incorrect.

 I CAN HINT: This question is evaluating the NCLEX® activity "*Participate in client consent process.*" "**CONSENT**" will assist you in organizing how to remember this concept. Remember it is the process whereby the client is informed of the risks, benefits, and alternatives of certain procedures and gives consent for a procedure to be done. Also note, that there can be a withdrawal of the consent either written or verbal, and can occur any time, even after the procedure has begun. "**LIFE**" will assist you in remembering the exceptions for the informed consent.

Client competency is why nurse witnesses signature, validate the signature, ensure consent is voluntary

Omit witnessing if client does not have all of the information to make an informed decision

Note client understands the benefits and risks of the procedure

Signed while client is free from mind-altering drugs or conditions; consent is a legal document

Educated on alternatives to procedure

Notes the healthcare provider performing the procedure

Taught procedure to the client in terms she/ he can understand

Exceptions for client to sign: "**LIFE**"

Life-threatening emergencies or urgent situations

Individuals are mentally incapacitated; Consent required of legal guardian or person specified to be medical of attorney.

For clients up to age 18, a parent's signature is generally required for consent.

Emancipated minor: Definition may vary, but usually this is a minor who is self-supporting and living away from home.

10.3 ③ Option #3 is correct. This will assist in maintaining correct alignment following surgery. The other options (#1, #2, and #4) are incorrect, and will not provide safe care following a hip replacement. After surgery the repaired hip should not flex greater than 90 degrees, and adduction and/or internal rotation of the extremity should be avoided. Excessive flexion and adduction may dislocate the hip prosthesis.

10.4 ① Option #1 is correct. Standard precautions are the appropriate type of infection precautions for hepatitis A. Hepatitis A is transmitted by the oral-fecal route. Option #2 is incorrect. Contact precautions, which is described in this option, are not necessary. The methods provided by standard precautions are the recommended standard of practice. Option #3 is not correct for this client. Option #4 is incorrect since this first part of the option indicates that this is transmitted by blood and blood products and airborne droplets, and this is not true. Hepatitis B and C are bloodborne.

I CAN HINT: CDC is the national organization that leads the research and implements the standards of care for the different infection control policies. Online resources: www.cdc. gov; www.nlm.nih.gov/medlineplus/ infectioncontrol.html

10.5 ② Option #2 is correct. The wheelchair should be positioned on the left side of the client, since the "strong side should lead" in order to provide safe nursing care. Options #1, #3, and #4 include correct plans of care and, therefore, would not mandate further intervention by the LPN.

10.6 ② The correct answer is option #2. Elderly adults may have difficulty swallowing. The HCP needs to be notified to change the order. Option #1 is incorrect. Some antibiotics cannot be given with milk and should not be crushed. The question was not specific enough to select this as an answer. Option #3 is incorrect since the elixir may require a dose change and this should be prescribed by the HCP not the pharmacist. Option #4 is incorrect because this may result with the client choking.

10.7 ② Option #2 is the correct answer. Elevation of the HOB allows easier breathing by. Option #1 is incorrect. Even if the client did require suctioning, the appropriate position would be to elevate the HOB versus to position them in the supine position. Option #3 is incorrect. There is no indication the client needs oxygen at this time. Even if the client did need oxygen, positioning would still be the priority for this question. Option #4 is incorrect for this question. While it may be important for the nurse to assess the lung sounds, it is not the priority for a client who is gasping in the middle of the night. Elevation of the HOB still remains the immediate priority.

10.8 ① Option #1 is the correct answer. Clients with diabetes mellitus have a problem with hyperglycemia. If a medication is ordered such as MethylPrednisolone Dose Pack that my elevate the blood sugar, then it is very important to monitor the serum glucose since the drug may work in opposition with the treatment for diabetes mellitus. Option #2 is incorrect. This does not answer the concern with the drug and disease. Option #3 is incorrect. While these packs may result in GI irritation, it is not addressing the question. Option #4 is incorrect. Vital signs are not answering the question.

10.9 ① Option #1 is the correct answer. A significant difference should be reported to the charge nurse. Option #2 is incorrect since there is an elevation in the blood pressure and it needs further evaluation. While option #3 is correct and needs to be document, it is not a priority at this time. Option #4 would be note worthy, but not priority.

10.10 ④ Option #4 is the correct answer. Amlopdipine (Norvasc) is a calcium channel blocker. It blocks calcium access to the cells causing a decrease in contractility, thus resulting in a decrease in the blood pressure. Option #1 is incorrect since it has no action on the respiratory rate. Options #2 and #3 are incorrect for this drug category.

10.11 ② Option #2 is correct answer. This client mandates immediate assessment since there may be a need to initiate CPR if there is not pulse or respirations. Option #1, #3, #4 are not a priority over option #2.

10.12 ③ Option #3 is the correct answer. These clinical findings definitely indicate a complication with hypoglycemia. (*Remember: "Hot and dry blood sugar is high, cold and clammy means you need some candy!"*) It is imperative that client receives the milk to assist with the complication of hypoglycemia. Option # 1 is incorrect. This does not address the complication presented by the client. Option #2 is incorrect. Insulin would further drive the blood sugar down. This would be inappropriate nursing care and would indicate a lack of understanding regarding the Standard of Practice for clients with hypoglycemia. Option #4 is incorrect. Intervention is a priority to increase the blood sugar prior to this action of notifying the HCP.

10.13 ④ Option #4 is correct. These 2 drugs may have an interaction that results in bleeding. Other drugs that may interact with warfarin (Coumadin) and result in bleeding may also include: garlic, ginger, ginseng, chamomile, etc. Option #1 is incorrect. Even though #1 may be attractive, this is not a nursing responsibility! Option #2 may be an accurate statement, but does not address the question regarding the client taking warfarin (Coumadin). Option #3 is also important, but not a priority over #4.

10.14 ③ Option #3 is the correct answer. This drug is excreted by the kidneys and may result in nephrotoxicity if there is any complications with the renal system. The BUN and creatinine should be assessed prior to initiating this order and continue to be monitored while taking the medication. Option #1 is an incorrect statement. Option # 2 is incorrect. Option #4 is an appropriate nursing action due to the infection, but is not a priority over #3.

10.15 ④ Option #4 is the correct answer and provides a legal explanation as to the reason the nurse is unable to respond to the mother's request. Option #1 is incorrect. Since the client is 21 years old, the HCP is not legally able to provide information to the mother without the consent of the son. Option #2 is avoiding responsibility. Option #3 is an accurate statement, but is a more adversarial statement than option #4.

10.16 ① Options #1, #2, #3, #4, are correct for
② this procedure. Option #5 is incorrect
③ since sterile gloves and bandaging were
④ used.

10.17 ④ Option #4 is most appropriate and reliable. Other acceptable ways to identify the client who does not have on an arm band may include: driver's license or a picture ID, phone number recall (if client alert), or have a client repeat and state name if client is alert and oriented and is not a very young child. Since this client is delusional, it is imperative to have a safe strategy for client identification. Stating name in this situation would not be appropriate. Options #1, #2 and #3 may not be reliable for this client, who is elderly and delusional.

10.18 ② Option #2 is correct answer. Contact isolation is the appropriate isolation protocol for clients with Clostridium Difficile. Option #1 is incorrect. This is not a sporicidal and should not be used when coming in contact with client with Clostridium Difficile. Option # 3 is incorrect. These clients should NEVER be in the same room. Option #4 is incorrect. Mask is not part of contact precautions unless the client is going to be suctioned or handling blood that is spurting, etc. The nurse should wear gloves and gown with this client and if the gloves are soiled during care, then these must be changed immediately.

10.19 ② Option #2 is the correct answer. An intramuscular injection requires a 1 to 1½ inch needle. The Bicillin is thick and will not easily go through the 25 gauge. Option #1 is incorrect because the needle is too long. Options #3 and #4 are incorrect because the gauge of the needle is too small.

10.20 ① Options #1, #2, #3, #5 are correct
② options for this pregnant client.
③ Option #4, turning the client to the left
⑤ side and providing only a small amount of oxygen are unlikely to assist with this emergency situation.

10.21 ① Options # 1, #3, and #5 are correct
③ options. Option #2 may be comforting,
⑤ but also may make client feel there is an expectation that client will fall. Option #4 is likely to cause accidents.

10.22 ① Option #1 is always a priority for any client experiencing a seizure. Option #2 is not a priority over airway patency. Option #3 is not appropriate for this condition. Option #4 is important to implement to assist the client from falling, but if there is any airway patency issue this will mandate intervention. The nurse will not just wait until seizure is finished if client is experiencing an obstructed airway.

10.23 ① Options #1, #2, #3, #4 are correct.
② Option #5 is incorrect since a full
③ assessment must be made prior to
④ reporting to the police.

10.24 Answer: 0.4mL, Available is 5 mg / mL and order is to administer 2mg. 5 mg in 1 mL, so 2 mg = 0.4 mL. Problem set up is: 5:1 = 2: X. Then cross multiply. 5X = 2. To solve for X divide each side of the equation by 5:

$$\frac{5X}{5} = \frac{2}{5}$$
$$X = 0.4$$

10.25 ② Option #2 is correct answer. It is important to avoid sudden movement of the head and to avoid unnecessary nursing procedures. Room should be dimly lit and quiet. Option #1 is incorrect. The diet should be a low-sodium or low-salt diet. Option #3 is incorrect since the room should be quiet

with minimal stimulation. Option #4 is incorrect since client should be on bed rest during an acute episode due to safety reasons. Client would be high risk for falling.

10.26 ③ Option # 3 is correct answer. Option #1 is incorrect since the specimen should not be collected from the drain. Option #2 is incorrect since the time of day is not relevant for a culture and sensitivity. Option #4 is not necessary for this procedure.

10.27 ③ Option #3 is the correct procedure. All other options are inappropriate for a child of this age. Injections should be administered in the vastus lateralis until the gluteus maximus is well developed, and this typically occurs after the child has been walking for 1 year.

10.28 Answer: 125 mL / hour. The nurse would divide the amount of fluid – 1000 mL by the number of hours – 8 – which is the infusion time for the IV fluid. 1000 / 8 = 125 mL / hour. Pumps are set at the rate per hour to infuse.

10.29 ② Option #2 is correct. Clean gloves should be worn at all times when handling any client's body / body fluids. Option #1 is incorrect because it is only secondary to wearing a pair of clean gloves. Option #3 is incorrect because it may take a longer time to stop bleeding due to possibility of coagulation being altered due to impaired liver. Option #4 is incorrect because needles should never be recapped due to safety and risk of unnecessary needle sticks.

10.30 ③ Correct order is: 3, 1, 4, 2, 5, 6
①
④
②
⑤
⑥

10.31 ④ Option #4 is correct answer. Mild to moderate rashes are the most common side effects of Bactrim. Options #1, #2, #3 are not side effects of Bactrim.

10.32 ④ Option # 4 is correct answer. This will increase the circulation and will decrease the risk of developing thrombophlebitis. Option #1 is incorrect because this will increase the risk by allowing blood to pool behind knee resulting in an increase risk for the development of thrombophlebitis. Option #2 is inappropriate. Option #3 is incorrect. It would be important to implement these actions while on bedrest; however, this answer does not address the question regarding the thrombophlebitis. It addresses potential pulmonary complications.

10.33 ③ Option #3 is correct. The Muslim culture believes that the same sex should provide care after death. Option #1 is incorrect since the Muslim culture grieves at home. Option #2 is inappropriate. Option #4 is incorrect since cremation is not practiced in the Muslim culture.

10.34 ② Option #2 is correct. The therapeutic level for digoxin is 0.5-2.0 ng/mL. This level is toxic 2.2 ng / mL. The medication should be held. Option #1 is incorrect since it should not be given with this level. Option #3 is an incorrect nursing action for this client. Option # 4 is incorrect since the blood level of digoxin is the priority.

10.35 ② Option #2 is correct due to safety issues. Options #1, #3, # 4 are not going to hurt anyone

10.36 ④ Option #4 is correct answer. The nurse should stand in front of the hearing impaired client. Option #1 is inappropriate for this situation because it is assuming the hearing loss is secondary to a build-up of wax. Option #2 is inappropriate for this situation. A sensory impaired client should always be aware that someone is present before being touched. Option #3 does not answer the question.

10.37 ② Option #2 is correct. This is a priority when establishing a bladder or bowel retraining program. Option #1 is not correct since the schedule should be

consistent and on a routine schedule versus a flexible schedule. While options #3 and #4 are part of the program, they are not a priority over option #2.

10.38 ① Option #1 is the correct procedure. Options #2, #3, #4 are not accurate procedures for collecting a throat culture.

10.39 ① Option #1 is correct answer. Daily weights are the most appropriate and most measurable in determining the client's state of hydration. While options #2, #3, #4 are included in the assessment for evaluating hydration, they are not as measurable and objective regarding client's hydration as the daily weight.

10.40 ④ Option #4 is correct since nitroglycerin (Nitrostat) can cause hypotension. Clients should avoid changing positions quickly to decrease the risk of falling. Option #1 is incorrect. The nitroglycerin (Nitrostat) should be taken with the onset of pain. Option #2 is incorrect. A burning sensation or stinging sensation indicates the medication is working. Option #3 is incorrect. Nitroglycerin (Nitrostat) is sublingual and should not be swallowed.

10.41 ② Option #2 is correct. Option #2 is a priority with medication administration down the nasogastric tube. Verification of tube placement prevents the instillation of medications into the lungs which may result in aspiration pneumonia. While options #1, #3, #4 may be appropriate nursing interventions, they are not specific to the question regarding the priority nursing action prior to administering meds through a nasogastric tube and are not a priority over option #2.

10.42 ② Option # 2 is correct. Sinequan is an antidepressant and signs of overdose include excitability and tremors. The other signs indicate depression which is the reason client is receiving this medication. Options #1, #3, #4 are not signs of Sinequan overdose.

 I CAN Publishing®, INC.

10.43 ② Option #2 is correct. It is a convenient method for administering medications to an infant. Options #1 and #3 are incorrect. Infant may not take all of formula, so is usually not added to the bottle. Option #4 is incorrect due to the position of the infant. The supine position may increase risk for aspiration.

10.44 ④ Option #4 is an undesirable effect from furosemide (Lasix). All other options are desired outcomes of the drug.

10.45 ② Option #2 is correct. The permit must be signed prior to receiving pre-op meds. Client is considered incapacitated after receiving narcotics. Options #1, #3, #4 are incorrect.

10.46 ② Option #2 is correct. If the pulse rate drops below the set rate on the pacemaker, then the pacer is malfunctioning. The pulse should be maintained at a minimal rate set on the pacemaker. Options #1 and #3 do not indicate malfunction of the pacemaker. Option # 4 may be early sign of infection at site, but does not indicate a pacemaker dysfunction.

10.47 ① Option #1 is correct. Hypovolemia from bleeding is most likely the cause of the symptoms and should be assessed prior to contacting the healthcare provider. Option #2 is controversial, and is not a priority over bleeding assessment. Option #3 should have some additional assessments prior to contacting the healthcare provider. Option #4 is incorrect since pain is an unlikely cause of the symptoms of shock.

10.48 ④ Option #4 is correct. This assessment is evaluating the spinal accessory nerve (number 11). All other options are for different cranial nerves. Option # 1 would be evaluating the hypoglossal nerve (number 12). Option #2 would be evaluating the first cranial nerve which is the olfactory nerve. Option #3 would be evaluating the 2nd cranial nerve which is the optic nerve.

10.49 ① ② ③ ④ Options #1, #2, #3 , #4 are correct. The assessment did not indicate a broken area of skin and does not need to be isolated as indicated in Option #5.

10.50 ① Option #1 is the best option provided. This situation provides a legal dilemma and should be addressed immediately. Options #2, #3, #4 are inappropriate for this situation.

10.51 Answer is: 25 gtts / minute. The nurse should divide 150 mL / hour by 60 minutes to get 2.5 mL / minute. Then multiply 2.5 mL / minute by 10 gtts / mL to get 25 gtts / minute at the rate to set the infusion set.

10.52 ③ Option #3 is the correct answer. This client is elderly; however, there is no indication that mobility is impaired. The greatest concern in evacuation is to move the largest number of clients initially, so those who are least critical are evacuated first. Option #1 has a client that has undergone major surgery, and is likely to be unable to ambulate due to anesthesia, and have an IV line in place. Option # 2 is a client who is 6 hours post-op following an appendectomy. Option #4 is a client that would also have an IV line in place, and would not be able to ambulate independently.

Disaster "ABC" = Ambulatory, Bedridden, Critical Care.

10.53 ② Option #2 is correct. Aspirating the syringe with a subcutaneous heparin solution can cause bruising. Option #1 is incorrect. When administering Heparin, the site should not be massaged after administration. Options #3 and #4 are incorrect. Heparin is usually administered subcutaneously with a 5/8-inch needle into the abdomen.

10.54 ② ④ ③ ① The correct sequence for donning PPE is options #2, #4, #3, #1.

10.55 ② Option #2 is the correct option. Oxygen is highly flammable and clients who have oxygen in the home are at risk for a fire if an open flame is present. Options #1 and #3 are incorrect. Option #4 is a normal finding in a client with COPD.

10.56 ② Option #2 is correct. There is no interpretation of events, only a description of what was found. Options #1 and #3 imply the reasoning for the event, which does not belong on the incident report. Option #4 uses the word "approximately", which leaves the documentation open for interpretation.

10.57 ② Option #2 is the correct option. It would be appropriate for a nutritional consultation for the family. This may decrease some of the anxiety. Option #1 is false reassurance. Option #3 does not address the specific problem. Option #4 is not within the scope of practice for the LPN.

10.58 ④ Option #4 is the correct answer. Options #1, #2, and #3, do not resolve or identify the conflict, and are punitive in nature. The role of the manager is to encourage positive relationships between the staff. In order to do that, the nurse needs to determine the source of conflict, and take action from there. Issues between staff members should always occur in a private setting.

10.59 ④ Option #4 is the correct answer. It is important to always begin antibiotics prior to any dental surgery or care. While options # 1 and #2 may be appropriate based on appropriate circumstances, they are not a priority over option # 4. Option #3 is an incorrect statement.

10.60 ④ Option #4 is the correct option. The nurse is signing as a legal witness, and without observing the client actually sign the form, the nurse is an illegal witness. Option #1 tells the physician the consent was signed, but does not address the legal issue. Options #2 and #3 do not serve the role of a legal witness.

10.61 ② Option #2 is the correct option. This client is presenting with heart failure and needs to conserve energy and oxygen. This client should not be up ambulating with the medical condition. Option #1 is correct practice to prevent causing any open lesions in mouth. Option #3 is also correct practice because this medication may result in GI irritation if not taken with food. Option #4 is correct practice. There is no need for the LPN to intervene with this nursing action. The UAP does not have the knowledge to understand the interpretation of the vital signs. This communication is a safe strategy.

10.62 ④ ⑤ Options # 4, and #5 are correct. These are part of contact precautions which is the requirement for Clostridium Difficile. Option #1 does not comply with isolation needed. Option #2 is inadequate hand cleansing for this organism since alcohol is not sporicidal. Option #3 is incorrect since a mask is not required.

10.63 ③ Option #3 is the best option. A written schedule with built-in extra time will allow the client to understand what is expected, and will allow her to participate at a slower pace. Options #1, #2, and #4 will not increase the client's independence and may interfere with client's self-esteem.

10.64 ③ Option #3 is correct. These assessment findings may indicate a complication with infection which requires a change in the plan of care for this client to prevent major complications with sepsis. Options #1, #2, #4 are not problems, and are not important to give in a report.

10.65 ④ Option #4 is the best option. It addresses the question regarding nursing care prior to admission for a client with seizure disorder. It is important to have the appropriate equipment at the bedside prior to the client being admitted. Option # 1 is incorrect because this would be completed after client was on the unit versus prior to admission. Option #2 is incorrect because it is not within the scope of practice for the LPN / VN to develop a plan of care in isolation of the

RN. Option #3 is incorrect since it is not a standard of practice to use padded tongue depressors.

10.66　① Option #1 is correct. It is within the scope of practice for the LPN to assess the breath sounds for this client. Option #2 is incorrect for the LPN since client is presenting with new symptoms of chest pain. This needs further assessment and analysis. Option #3 is incorrect since client needs further analysis to determine a need to revise plan for oxygen delivery. Option #4 is incorrect because the LPN cannot develop a plan in isolation of the RN. This must be done collaboratively.

10.67　④ Option #4 is correct. This may indicate the client has an intracranial bleed. It is important to follow up with this clinical finding. Option #1 is incorrect since this is the reason the client is receiving the medication. This is not a complication from the drug; it is a complication from the DVT. Option #2 may happen, but is not a priority over a potential intracranial hemorrhage. Option #3 is not the correct lab report for this medication. The pTT would be evaluated for a client taking heparin.

10.68　④ Option #4 is correct. This "high pressure alarm" indicates there is either water in the tubing or client needs suctioning. Client could also be lying on or biting on the tubing which may result in the "high pressure alarm" going off. During this process, it is always important to evaluate the reading on the pulse oximeter to determine the effect on the client. Option #1 is incorrect because the immediate action should be focused on the client. Option #2 does not address the challenge with the alarm. Oxygen will not correct the "high pressure alarm" and / or correct the cause with the client that is contributing to this challenge. Option #3 is incorrect practice. Alarms should NEVER be silenced.

Remember: "**High**" rhymes with **DRY** and "Low" has an L in it to remember **LEAK**. This will help you always remember the meaning of ventilator alarms and help you answer questions successfully!!

10.69　①⑤ Options #1 and# 5 are correct because they require general nursing care that is congruent with the LPN Nurse Practice Act. Option # 2 would require IV management and specialized assessment skills. Option # 3 would require initial assessment. LPNs can do ongoing assessments, but it is not in the scope of practice to complete the initial assessment. Option #4 is incorrect, because it requires initial teaching. The LPN can reinforce teaching, but it is currently not in the scope of practice to do the initial teaching.

10.70　③ Option #3 is the correct answer. The nurse needs to see the client who is retaining CO_2 and is experiencing respiratory acidosis. The restlessness may be indicative of hypoxia and with the elevation in the heart rate, the client is experiencing some significant changes. Options #1, #2, and #4 are not a priority over #3. Option #1 reflects clinical findings WNL. Option #2 is a finding that needs to be monitored closely, but is not a priority over option #3. Option #4 is resting and is not a priority over #3.

10.71　①②④⑤ Options # 1, #2, #4, #5 are correct. The transfusion should be started with a #18 – #19 gauge needle.

10.72　④ Option #4 is the correct option. This statement clearly indicates that the caregiver is attempting to get the client to discuss thoughts and feelings. Option #1 is inappropriate, since this is not helping the client to deal with feelings. Option #2 is inappropriate and very non-therapeutic. This will not allow client to process feelings. Option #3 is false reassurance and is also non-therapeutic.

Remember: "**TRUST**" will assist you in remembering therapeutic communication: Try expression, Reflection of words, Use of Silence, Set Limits, Time with client

10.73　③ Option #3 is the correct answer. This situation projects hopelessness, insomnia, and physical changes with the weight loss. This is definitely a priority to report to get additional support for wife prior to any additional complications. Option #1 is not a priority, since she recognizes the need to get help. Option #3 (the correct answer) does not indicate this self-awareness. Option #2 is a great thing to happen. This indicates she has support and is not trying to do this alone. Option #4 also reflects self-awareness, and is a healthy behavior.

10.74 ② Option #2 is the best answer. Listening has the highest priority. Further assessment is needed prior to #1 and #3. Option #4 is not honoring the grief.

10.75 ④ Option #4 is very important as extravasation of this drug can cause necrosis. Options #1 and #2 are not priority. Option #3 is incorrect because Phenergan has no analgesic properties.

10.76 ① Options #1 and #2 are the correct
       ② answers. Option #3 is incorrect since the ear irrigation is not likely to increase intracranial pressure. Option #4, the provider does not need to be called at this point. Option #5 can be dangerous as the ear wax can be pushed further down in the ear canal and damage the drum.

10.77 ① Option#1 is the correct answer. If the client has claustrophobia, the scan may cause severe anxiety. Option #2 is incorrect as aspirin is not utilized in a CAT scan. Options #3 and #4 are unnecessary assessment data needed for this exam.

10.78 ② Option #2 is incorrect. This reflex normally disappears between 3-4 months. All other options are normal at this age.

10.79 ③ Option #3 is the correct answer. The arms should be bent, so that the weight is placed on the hands and arms. Option #1 can damage the nerve under the arm. Option #2 is incorrect because crutches should be placed 8-10 inches in front of each step. Option #4 may be unsafe.

10.80 ② Options #2 and #5 are correct.
       ⑤ Allergies come from egg, foul, and neomycin. Immunizations must also be age appropriate. Options #1 and #3 are incorrect. There is no absolute relationship between family members and allergies and reactions. Option #4 is more significant for oral polio immunization.

10.81 ③ Option #3 is correct. If the client is allergic to latex, all other options are inappropriate.

10.82 ① Option #1 is correct answer. All other options are secondary to this one. Option #4 should have been assessed prior to surgery.

10.83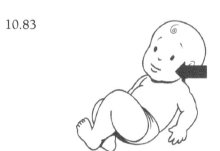

10.84 ② Option #2 is correct because this is when the breasts are least engorged. Option #1 is when the breasts are most engorged. Option #3 is unnecessary and Option #4 is for post-menopausal women.

10.85 ① Option #1 is correct as epigastric pain is usually indicative of an impending seizure or possible eclampsia. Options #2 and #3 are expected observations during pregnancy. Option #4 should be addressed, but is not priority to #1.

10.86 ① Option #1 is correct. These assessment findings may be a result of diabetes insipidus, especially since the clues were provided in the stem with the signs of thirst and fatigue. Diabetes insipidus results from a deficiency of antidiuretic hormone (ADH), also known as vasopressin, secreted by the posterior lobe of the pituitary lobe of the pituitary gland (neurohypophysis). Decreased ADH reduces the ability of the distal and collecting renal tubules in the kidneys to concentrate urine, resulting in excessive diluted urination, excessive thirst, and excessive fluid intake. Other assessments may include: weight loss, muscle weakness, headache, tachycardia, hypotension, poor skin turgor, dry mucous membranes, constipation, and dizziness. This may result from cranial surgery, irradiation, or from a defect in the hypothalamus or pituitary gland. This may also be drug-induced. Option #2 is incorrect. This is appropriate behavior and safe post-op care, so this does not need to be reported. Option #3 is not a priority over option #1. Option #4 does not address the question. The specific gravity does indicate the urine is concentrated, but does not provide any additional information indicating the client has SIADH, and this does NOT reflect the current assessments of thirst and fatigue which are provided in the stem of the question

10.87 ① Options #1,#2, #3 are correct answers.
② Options #4 and #5 include foods high
③ in residue.

10.88 ② Option #2 should be tried first. This is the least invasive, and if it works all other options will not be necessary. Option #4 is incorrect and irrigation should never be forced.

10.89 ② Option #2 is the correct answer. As the onset of action for Humalog is short, less than one hour. This assessment indicates the client is hypoglycemic. Foods such as milk and crackers will usually correct these symptoms. Options #1 and #4 delay the appropriate intervention. Option #3 is unnecessary unless the client is unconscious.

10.90 ② Option #2 is correct. This would allow the client to cry or express anger or fear. Other options do not allow for immediate expression of reaction to this crisis.

10.91 ④ Option #4 is correct since artificial nails are not allowed with direct client care. Options # 1, #2 and #3 do not require further teaching. These indicate an understanding of infection control through appropriate hand washing.

10.92 ③ Option #3 is correct. Angina presents with depressed ST segment. A client with an MI (myocardial infarction) would most likely experience an elevation in the ST segment on the cardiac monitor. Option #1 is incorrect. This change would occur with an elevation in the potassium level. Option #2 is incorrect because it would occur with an MI. Option #4 is incorrect because this would occur as a result of a heart block versus angina.

10.93 ④ Option #4 is correct. This option indicates a potential risk for infection. The other options are desired for this client.

10.94 ② Option #2 is correct. This option is an objective assessment to evaluate the nursing action. Option #1 is not the priority over #2 for this client with a tracheostomy. Option #3 is incorrect. This is the responsibility of the nurse. Option #4 is incorrect because it is subjective versus option #2 which is an objective evaluation.

10.95 ① Option #1 is the correct answer. The client is bleeding and mandates immediate intervention by initiating pressure over the incision site to stop the bleeding. Option #2 is incorrect. The client is bleeding, so assessment of pulses is not appropriate until pressure is applied. Options #3 and #4 are incorrect, and do not address the question.

NOTES

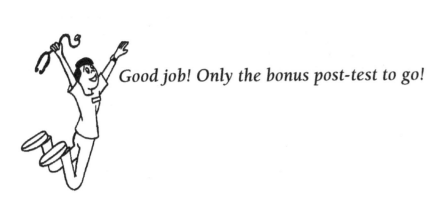 *Good job! Only the bonus post-test to go!*

NOTES

CHAPTER 11

Bonus Post-Test

*It's the action, not the fruit of the action that's
important. You have to do the right thing. . . You may
never know what results come from your action,
but if you do nothing, there will be no result.*
—Gandhi

✔ **Clarification of this test ...**

Just keep on working on your testing practice and study. Here are more questions to
help you identify your study needs.

11.1 Which nursing plan of action indicates the
UAP understands how to safely care for a
client with Peripheral Artery Disease?

① Measure the diameter of the calf of the
leg and compare to unaffected leg.
② Position the affected leg above the level
of the heart.
③ Apply compression stockings after client
gets out of bed.
④ Assist client to dangle legs off the side of
the bed.

11.2 Which action by the LPN/LVN indicates
the need for the nurse to intervene
immediately?

① The LPN/LVN brings breakfast to
a client who is scheduled for an
echocardiogram later in the morning.
② The LPN/LVN assesses a client's
blood pressure prior to administering
nitroglycerin (Nitor-Stat) 0.4 mg SL.
③ The LPN/LVN assists a client to
the bathroom 20 minutes after the
client has returned from a coronary
arteriogram.

④ The LPN/ LVN returns a client to bed
after the heart rate increases from 72 to
100 while ambulating in the hall.

11.3 The LPN/LVN is the charge nurse in a long-
term care facility and is developing a quality
assurance program in collaboration with the
nursing director for ongoing assessments of
all residents with a diagnosis of Congestive
Heart Failure. Which of these nursing
actions should be included in the plan that
would be most appropriate for delegation to
another LPN/LVN team leader?

① Assess breath sounds and check for
edema daily.
② Check charts to make certain clients are
receiving verapamil (Calan) as ordered.
③ Review all medications with the client
every other day.
④ Weigh all residents monthly.

11.4 Which of these clients should be seen immediately after shift report?

① A client presenting with a blood pressure of 150/90 and resting quietly.
② A client presenting with +1 pitting edema in ankles.
③ A client complaining of pain in calf of right leg when walking but subsides when stops walking.
④ A client awakening with dyspnea, severe anxiety, jugular vein distention (JVD), and frothy pink sputum.

11.5 A client is being treated for hypovolemia. Which observation would the nurse identify as the expected outcome to fluid replacement?

① Arterial pH 7.34.
② Blood pressure increase from 108/68 to 126/80.
③ Specific gravity–1.030.
④ Urine output 160 mL/5 hours.

11.6 Which assessment best indicates proper rehydration for a client presenting with vomiting and diarrhea?

① 400 mL of po intake over 3 hours.
② Heart rate of 105 per minute.
③ Respiratory rate of 32 per minute.
④ Urine output of 100 mL per hour.

11.7 Which documentation indicates an understanding of how to position a client who is experiencing fluid overload from too much IV fluid and is presenting with dyspnea, R–38, HR–120, extremely anxious, and crackles throughout lung fields.

① Client positioned in the High-Fowler's position.
② Client positioned in the Lithotomy position.
③ Client positioned in the Low-Fowler's position.
④ Client positioned in the Sim's position.

11.8 Which nursing action would require intervention from the charge nurse with a nurse who is performing tracheostomy care for a client?

① The nurse removes old dressings and cleans off excess secretions.
② The nurse replaces the inner cannula and cleans the stoma site.
③ The nurse uses universal precaution when cleaning the inner cannula.
④ The nurse secures new ties in place prior to removing old ties.

11.9 Which assignment would be most appropriate for a new nurse of 8 months who is pulled from the surgical unit to the medical unit?

① A 40-year-old client with SARS and is on airborne precautions.
② A 50-year-old client following thoracic surgery and is on a ventilator.
③ A 60-year-old client who just returned from a bronchoscopy.
④ A 70-year-old client who needs teaching regarding the use of an incentive spirometer.

11.10 The nurse is caring for a client who is two days post-op abdominal surgery. Which assessment data, on the following intake and output sheet (I&O), would require further action by the nurse?

Source	7 A.M.–7 P.M.	7 P.M.–7 A.M.
P. O.	0 mL	0 mL
IV	1500 mL	1500 mL
Urine	900 mL	1000 mL
Nasogastric tube	500 mL	50 mL

① P. O. intake
② Intravenous fluid balance
③ Urine output
④ Nasogastric suction drainage

11.11 Which of these clinical findings would require further assessment and intervention for a client who is taking hydromorphone (Dilaudid) post-thoracic surgery?

① 0800—BP–110/78; 0900—BP–122/82.

② 0800—RR–18/min; 0900—RR–22/min.

③ 0800—Urine output–72 mL/hr; 0900—Urine output–40 mL/hr.

④ 0800—resting quietly, 0900–client talking and active.

11.12 Which of these actions by the UAP for a client with hypertension mandate intervention by the LPN/LVN?

① Provides client with a snack of a fresh fruit.

② Takes client to physical therapy to engage in regular exercise program.

③ Takes the blood pressure with a cuff that is one third the size of the upper arm.

④ Weighs client daily using the same scales.

11.13 A client is being treated with Lorazepam (Ativan) 5 mg IV q hour. Which nursing action would be priority after administration?

① Have naloxone (Narcan) at the bedside and ready for administration.

② Obtain a baseline pulse oximetry reading.

③ Do a complete neurological exam every shift.

④ Check respiratory status every 15 minutes.

11.14 What statement from family members of an 80-year-old client receiving morphine prior to coming to the unit, would the LPN / LVN assess to indicate they need additional reinforcement of the teaching regarding the client's progress?

① "We understand that due to our mom's age she will be monitored closely for any changes in clinical condition."

② "We understand that she will respond and wake up like she did 20 years ago after receiving the morphine."

③ "We understand that we need to provide safety precautions for her at home due to her sensory limitations."

④ "We understand that due to the physiological changes that may occur with age that her heart and lungs may have more complications due to the decrease in physiologic reserve."

11.15 The nurse indicates a safe understanding of infection control standards for a client with SARS when putting on which of the PPE prior to suctioning? *Select all that apply.*

① N 95 mask

② Gloves

③ Gown

④ shoe covers

⑤ hair net

11.16 Which system-specific assessment would be the priority for the LPN to report to the charge nurse for a client with congestive heart failure?

① R–18 increased to R–22 with exertion.

② HR–72 decreased from 88 after taking digoxin (Lanoxin).

③ Weight increase from 142 lbs to 146 lbs in 48 hours.

④ Oxygen saturation decreased from 98% to 95% with exertion.

11.17 Twenty-four hours after abdominal surgery, which plan would be a priority to prevent complications of flatulence?

① Assist the client to walk in the hall every 2 hours.

② Encourage the client to do leg exercises in bed.

③ Encourage the client to drink carbonated beverages daily.

④ Instruct the client to turn from side to side.

11.18 What intervention should the nurse implement prior to administering esomeprazole (Nexium)?

① Check for allergies to cephalosporins.
② Elevate the foot of the bed.
③ Verify identity of client with wrist bracelet and ask to state date of birth.
④ Order an infusion pump for the client.

11.19 Which information is important to include in the teaching plan for a client who will be taking antacids at home following discharge?

① Take antacids prior to meals.
② Take antacids with ranitidine (Zantac).
③ Take antacids 15 minutes after meals.
④ Take antacids 1 hour after meals.

11.20 Which statement from the client indicates an understanding of how to successfully take psyllium (Metamucil)?

① "I will take this medication with 1 oz. of water."
② "I will take this medication in the dry form."
③ "I will mix this medication in 8-10 oz. of water."
④ "I will decrease the fiber in my diet."

11.21 Which of these clients should be assessed immediately after report? A client presenting with:

① intermittent left lower abdominal pain.
② sour taste in mouth and dyspepsia.
③ heartburn, bloating and nausea.
④ sudden abdominal pain radiating throughout abdomen and absent bowel sounds.

11.22 A client has a nasogastric (NG) tube to low intermittent suction. The client is lying flat in bed and begins to cough and vomit. What would be the priority of care for this client?

① Notify the provider of care regarding the complication.

② Assess bowel sounds.
③ Insert 30 milliliters of Normal Saline to check the patency.
④ Reposition client to side.

11.23 A client diagnosed with cerebrovascular accident (CVA) is being discharged from the hospital. Which safety modification is appropriate to include in the discharge teaching?

① Position at a 90-degree angle for meals.
② Remove floor rugs.
③ Utilize low lighting.
④ Obtain a long-handled spoon for feedings.

11.24 Which roommate would be most appropriate for the LPN / LVN to assign for a 12-year-old client with first- and second-degree burns on the abdominal area and bilateral arms?

① A ten-year-old with meningitis.
② An eleven-year-old with methicillin-resistant staphaureus. (MRSA)
③ A twelve-year-old with second-degree burns to lower extremities with a T–102 degrees F and taking an antibiotic.
④ A thirteen-year-old who is post-op appendectomy.

11.25 A nurse has instructed a client with multiple sclerosis about risk factors for disease exacerbations. Which statement by the client indicates a need for further teaching?

① "I will incorporate periods of rest into my daily routine."
② "Practicing good hand hygiene may help me avoid contracting infections."
③ " I will enact safety measures to avoid physical injury."
④ "Bathing in hot water will alleviate symptom development."

11.26 A client with terminal cancer is nearing the end of life. Which plan would best meet the client's emotional needs?

① Provide the client with a room where family can be present.
② Make sure that the client has an advanced directive on the chart.
③ Consult the hospital chaplain or client's personal spiritual advisor.
④ Provide the client with a journal to record final thoughts for family and friends.

11.27 A psychiatric client with the diagnosis of schizophrenia tells the nurse that he is the President of the United States. What would be the priority action for the LPN / LVN?

① Confront the client regarding this delusion and bring back to reality.
② Reflect this statement back to the client to encourage therapeutic communication.
③ Respond with an open-ended response to get client to further discuss this thoughts.
④ Verify the identity of the client prior to administering the medications.

11.28 Which nursing action is of primary importance during the implementation of a behavior modification treatment program?

① Confirm that all staff members understand and comply with the treatment plan.
② Establish mutually-agreed-upon, realistic goals.
③ Ensure that the potent reinforcers (rewards) are important to the client.
④ Establish a fixed interval schedule for reinforcement.

11.29 Which statement indicates the client understands how to safely care for self following a vagotomy with antrectomy for treating a duodenal ulcer and preventing the development of dumping syndrome ?

① "I should eat a lot of carbohydrates."
② "I will drink fluids with my meals."
③ "I should lie down after I eat."
④ "I should remain upright after meals."

11.30 A client in the long term healthcare facility is going out with his daughter for the day. The LPN / LVN is reviewing the proper technique for using a cane. Which of these return demonstrations indicate the client understands how to use the cane safely?

① The client holds the cane on the affected side and moves it with the affected leg.
② The client holds the cane on the unaffected side and moves cane forward followed by affected side and then the unaffected leg.
③ The client holds the cane on the unaffected side and moves it with the unaffected leg followed by the affected side.
④ The client holds the cane on the affected side and moves it with the unaffected leg.

11.31 The LPN / LVN is monitoring a client who was admitted to the Neuro Unit with a diagnosis of a CVA. Which of the following clinical findings necessitates an immediate intervention by the LPN / LVN?

① Dilantin level of 15 mg/dl.
② Blood Pressure of 130/90 is now 155/92.
③ Pupils that were reactive at 4 mm and equal and now are 6 mm.
④ Change in posturing from abnormal flexion to abnormal extension.

11.32 What would the LPN / LVN include in the plan for a Hindu family who had a father who just died?

① Encourage family to chant at the bedside while performing the "Last Rites".
② Allow the family to wash the body after the father died.
③ Only allow the priest to touch the body after death.
④ Never ask for donation of the organs.

11.33 Which of these nursing actions indicate the LPN / LVN understands how to safely provide care for a client with Streptococcal (Group A) pharyngitis? The LPN / LVN wears:

① A gown when entering the room.
② Gloves when taking blood pressure.
③ A surgical mask when 5 feet from the client.
④ A surgical mask when 2 feet from the client.

11.34 Which of these personal protective measures should the LPN/LVN use when suctioning a client? *Select all that apply.*

① Double glove
② Gown
③ Gloves
④ Goggles
⑤ Shoe covers

11.35 Which of these nursing actions indicate the LPN/LVN understand how to safely administer nifedipine (Procardia)?

① Administers with grapefruit juice.
② Administers to client with a pulse of 56 BPM.
③ Instructs client to increase fiber and fluid intake.
④ Administers to a client in heart failure.

CATEGORY ANALYSIS – BONUS POST-TEST

1. Basic Care and Comfort
2. Coordinated Care
3. Reduction of Risk Potential
4. Coordinated Care
5. Basic Care and Comfort
6. Basic Care and Comfort
7. Physiological Adaptation
8. Coordinated Care
9. Coordinated Care
10. Physiological Adaptation
11. Pharmacological Therapies
12. Coordinated Care
13. Pharmacological Therapies
14. Health Promotion
15. Safety & Infection Control
16. Basic Care and Comfort
17. Basic Care and Comfort
18. Safety & Infection Control
19. Pharmacological Therapies
20. Pharmacological Therapies
21. Coordinated Care
22. Reduction of Risk Potential
23. Reduction of Risk Potential
24. Safety & Infection Control
25. Health Promotion
26. Psychosocial Integrity
27. Psychosocial Integrity
28. Psychosocial Integrity
29. Health Promotion
30. Basic Care and Comfort
31. Reduction of Risk Potential
32. Psychosocial Integrity
33. Safety & Infection Control
34. Safety & Infection Control
35. Pharmacological Therapies

DIRECTIONS

1. Determine questions missed by checking answers.
2. Write the number of the questions missed across the top line marked "item missed."
3. Check category analysis page to determine category of question.
4. Put a check mark under item missed and beside content.
5. Count check marks in each row and write the number in totals column.
6. Use this information to:
   • identify areas for further study.
   • determine which content test to take next.

We recommend studying content where most items are missed—then taking that content test.

Number of the Questions Incorrectly Answered

Pre-test	Items Missed																											Totals
C Coordinated Care																												
O Safety and Infection Control																												
N Health Promotion and Maintenance																												
T Psychosocial Integrity																												
E Physiological Integrity: Physiological Adaptation																												
N Physiological Integrity: Reduction of Risk																												
T Physiological Integrity: Basic Care and Comfort																												
Physiological Integrity: Pharmacological Therapies																												

I CAN Publishing®, INC.

ANSWERS & RATIONALES

11.1 ④ Option #4 is correct. This will assist in getting blood flowing to the lower extremities after being in bed. Option #1 would be appropriate for a concern with a DVT. Option #2 is incorrect. While elevation may be appropriate to reduce swelling, do not elevate above the level of the heart because extreme elevation slows arterial blood flow to the feet. Option #3 is incorrect for this client. Insulated socks, however, would be appropriate for this client to assist with promoting vasodilation. If the extremity gets cold, this will result in vasoconstriction which will further decrease the arterial blood flow to the extremity. Peripheral arterial disease (PAD) is characterized by inadequate flow of blood. Peripheral venous disease is a disease of the veins that interferes with adequate flow of blood from the extremities.

11.2 ③ Option # 3 is the correct answer. This client should remain in bed with the extremity straight based on the hospital protocol. This is inappropriate to get client up to bathroom within this short time frame. Options #1, #2, and #4 do not require the nurse to intervene immediately due to unsafe care.

11.3 ① Option #1 is correct answer. Clients with congestive heart failure need to be assessed for both edema and the breath sounds. Remember if the client is in right sided heart failure, think about "REST" of body which includes peripheral edema, increase in weight, hepatosplenomegaly (increase in abdominal girth), jugular vein distention (JVD). If it is left sided heart failure, remember left has an "L" for LUNGS. The client will present with pulmonary edema or any changes in the lungs such as with adventitious breath sounds. Option #2 is incorrect. If a client is in congestive heart failure, then this

medication most likely will not be given to all clients. Option # 3 is not necessary this frequently. Option #4 is incorrect. Clients must be weighed daily or at least on a routine basis versus monthly.

11.4 ④ Option #4 is correct. This client should be seen immediately, since the client is experiencing pulmonary edema and heart failure. Option #1 is a concern, but is not a priority over option #4 who is in acute distress. Option #2 is not a priority over option #4. Option #3 is a concern due to the complication with intermittent claudication (peripheral arterial disease), but is not an acute problem like option #4, so is not a priority in this situation.

11.5 ② Option #2 is the correct answer. This value indicates the volume has improved from the fluid replacement. Options #1, #3, and #4 are not correct for this situation. Option #3 would have a specific gravity of 1.012–1.015 if client was treated successfully. Option #4 is incorrect since client is only voiding 32 mL/hour which does not indicate client has a successful outcome from the fluid replacement.

11.6 ④ Option #4 is correct for this situation. Options #1, #2, and #3 are not correct for this question. Option # 1 does not indicate the output, and just because we know how much client took in, we have no idea how much client voided. Option #2 does not indicate proper rehydration because the rate is still too fast. Option #3 is incorrect.

11.7 ① Option #1 is correct. This position will assist with breathing for this client who is in fluid overload. Options #2, #3, and #4 are incorrect for this client's respiratory complications. These positions will not facilitate breathing like option #1.

11.8 ③ Option #3 is correct answer because the precautions should be surgical asepsis. Options #1, #2, and #4 do not require intervention by the charge nurse since these represent safe nursing practice.

11.9 ④ Option #4 is correct. Surgical clients require teaching on how to use the incentive spirometers. This nurse should have this common knowledge, and be able to support the client with this intervention. Options #1, #2, and #3 may not be appropriate for this nurse due to lack of experience, and not providing nursing care routinely for these type of clients.

11.10 ④ Option #4 is correct. Sudden cessation or drastic decrease of nasogastric drainage indicates blockage or disruption of the drainage system. Normal gastric production is 1-1.5 L daily. 500 ml per twelve-hour shift is expected. Option #1 is incorrect because the client has a draining nasogastric tube. P.O. intake is not expected. Option #2 demonstrates that the I.V. fluid balance is appropriate. Option #3 is incorrect because the urine output is slightly more than intake and is not a cause of concern.

11.11 ③ Option #3 is correct due to the risk with a decrease in the urine output as a result of this medication. The trend is going down and the nurse needs to intervene. Options #1, #2, and #4 are not a priority over option #3. Option #1 has gone up versus down. Option #2 has gone up versus down. Option #4 does not require any assessment based on the current assessments.

11.12 ③ Option #3 is the correct answer. The cuff should cover two thirds of the size of the upper arm. This current option may result in an inappropriate blood pressure value, so the LPN / LVN needs to intervene to provide accurate information on how to perform this procedure safely and effectively. Options #1, #2, and #4 include safe nursing practice and do not require intervention.

11.13 ④ Option #4 is correct. Benzodiazepines may cause respiratory depression, especially by IV route. Narcan is only for opioids. Option #2 would need to be accomplished BEFORE administration. Option #3 is incorrect because neuro exams need to be evaluated more frequently.

11.14 ② Option #2 is the correct answer. Older clients do not respond to medication like they did when they were younger due to changes in the pharmacokinetics. There is a decrease in the metabolism, absorption, distribution, and excretion with age. It may take client longer to wake up than it did 20 years ago when liver, renal, GI system and protein receptors were not decreased in functioning. Options #1, #3, and #4 indicate an appropriate understanding of the aging process.

11.15 ① ② ③ Options #1, #2, #3 are correct. There is no indication for options #4 and #5 for SARS.

11.16 ③ Option #3 is correct. Weight increase is one of the first assessment findings for clients with congestive heart failure. Options #1, #2, and #4 are not priorities over option #3.

11.17 ① Option #1 is the correct answer. Ambulation is an excellent intervention to prevent complications of flatulence. Options #2, #3, and #4 are not effective for this complication.

11.18 ③ Option #3 is the correct answer. The other options are incorrect.

11.19 ④ Option #4 is correct. Antacids should be taken 1 hour after meals in order to achieve optimum results for the antacids. Options #1, #2, and #3 are incorrect.

11.20 ③ Option #3 is correct. The client should mix the drug in 8-10 oz. of water; stir and drink immediately. Option #1 is incorrect. Actually, even though the drug is mixed with 8-10 oz of water, it should also be followed with 1 extra glass of water. Client should be instructed to drink a minimum of eight 8-oz. glasses of water per day. Option #2 is incorrect. Do not ever swallow in dry form. Option #4 is incorrect. Fiber should be increased in the diet.

11.21 ④ Option #4 is correct. These assessments may indicate a medical emergency. While the other options may need further assessment, they are not a priority over option #4.

11.22 ④ Option #4 is the priority for this client in order to prevent aspiration from the vomiting. Options #1, #2, #3 are not priorities over option #4. The immediate concern is to reposition to prevent aspiration.

11.23 ② Option #2 is appropriate due to the risk for falls. Options #1, #3, and #4 are not priorities over Option #2.

11.24 ④ Option #4 is most appropriate due to the decrease risk for developing an infection. Options #1, #2, and #3 would all present the risk for infection.

11.25 ④ Option #4 is correct. This could be unsafe for the client, so further teaching is required to assure client safety. Options #1, #2, and #3 do not indicate a need for further teaching since these would be included in safe client care.

11.26 ① Option #1 is correct. Providing a room for the client's family would be the best plan to meet the client's emotional needs. Option #2 does not meet the client's emotional needs. Option #3 is secondary. Option #4 is secondary.

11.27 ④ Option #4 is a priority due to safety. Option #1 is partially correct, but nurses do not confront this client. Options #2 and #3 are part of therapeutic communication and are not answering the question.

11.28 ① Option #1 is correct. To successfully implement a behavior modification plan, all staff members need to be included in the program development and to allow time for discussion of concerns from each nursing staff member. Consistency and follow-through is of utmost importance to prevent or diminish the level of manipulation by the staff or client during the implementation of this program. Options #2, #3, and #4 are important in designing an effective behavior modification program. Option #1, however, still remains the priority in order to achieve successful outcomes.

11.29 ③ Option #3 is the correct answer. Options #1, #2, and #4 are incorrect. These may contribute to complications from dumping syndrome.

11.30 ② Option #2 is correct. The cane acts is a support and assist in weight-bearing for the weaker leg. Option #1 should read the cane is held on the unaffected side. Option #3 should read that it moves and then the affected leg moves followed by the unaffected leg. Option #4 should read the can is held on unaffected side.

11.31 ④ Option #4 is correct. These changes in posturing may indicate the ominous sign of increased cerebral edema and potential herniation. Options #1, #2, and #3 are not a priority over #4.

11.32 ② Option #2 is correct for the Hindu family. For an Islamic family member's death, only relatives or a priest may touch the body. The family washes the body and then turns it to face Mecca. Option #1 is appropriate for a Buddhist family. Option #4 is not true. Donation of organs may be done.

11.33 ④ Option #4 is correct. The nurse should wear a mask when 3 feet from the client. Option #1 is not necessary for this client when entering the room. If the nurse was suctioning, responding to an emergency involving blood, cleaning an incontinent client with diarrhea, or irrigating a wound, then the gown would definitely be necessary. Option #2 is not necessary for this client. This would be important if the client needed contact isolation such as if they had MRSA, VRE, a major abscess, or a decubitus. Option #3 is incorrect for this client. The nurse needs to wear a mask if at least 3 feet of the client.

11.34 ② Options #2, #3, and #4 are correct.
③ They represent the universal / standard
④ precautions that must be followed when suctioning a client. Option #1 is not included in this standard. This should not be necessary if gloves are not damaged. Option #5 is not included in this standard and is not necessary when suctioning a client in universal / standard precautions.

11.35 ③ Option #3 is correct. There is a potential for constipation when taking this nifedipine (Procardia). Option #1 is not correct since grapefruit juice and grapefruit can cause increased levels and effects of the medication. Option #2 is not a priority over option #3. Procardia and calcium channel blockers may cause bradycardia due to the physiological effects on the heart of decreasing contractility by inhibiting the calcium transport into the myocardial and vascular smooth muscle cells. The provider of care will typically order the parameters of when to hold the medication. This typically is with a heart rate below 50 or 60 BPM. Of course, if the client is symptomatic due to bradycardia, then the medication should also be held. The provider of care should then be notified. Option #4 is incorrect. If a client is in heart failure, this medication may create more complications with the failure due to the action of the drug.

I CAN Publishing®, INC.